Reviews and comments on the first edition:

"*White Coat, Clenched Fist* is the account of one physician's political education and efforts to change the system. It is a first class piece of writing but is more important for what it says than for how it says it. I had the privilege of counting Fitzhugh among my students when he was in medical school, and our past paths touched again as he served medical organizations on the left and I on the right. Reading this book increased my respect for Mullan and made me aware that most of us do very little to improve the condition of those that society has placed at a disadvantage."

William R. Barclay, M.D., *Journal of the American Medical Association*

"Mullan writes vividly about his medical education and postdoctoral training. His descriptions of these experiences make a political point. He found medical education and the medical system bureaucratic and unyielding, much less concerned with shaping medical care to suit the communities and lifestyles of the poor than with preserving a comfortable form of private practice."

Norman E. Zinberg, *New York Times Book Review*

"Fitzhugh Mullan's honest, intelligent, and readable autobiography shows . . . that the radicalism of his generation did change America. . . . And it will be a disaster if younger generations look back on it as a picturesque aberration."

Godfrey Hodgson, *Washington Post Book Review*

"*White Coat, Clenched Fist* is an uncommon literary achievement. . . . Nowhere has the intrinsic behavior modifying function of medical education been more vividly drawn. . . . A rare man, a rare book."

Quentin D. Young, *Chicago Sun-Times*

"An important, intelligent, and superbly written new book . . . that is not a polemic. Throughout his young career Mullan has chosen to channel his anger at the system into deeds, not histrionics."

Robert Mayer, *Santa Fe Reporter*

"Mullan offers a firsthand view of the world the patient never sees—the grueling internships, the taboos of death and sex. Not content to take the money and run, Mullan became more dissatisfied with the medical profession when he began to practice. . . . Mullan made waves with the American Medical Association. He stirred what many would prefer to let go unnoticed with the admired, awesome medical profession."

Ginny Stolicker, *Oakland Press*

"Dr. Mullan's book is important because it raises some serious questions about the quality of medical care in the U.S. at a time when consumer groups as well as congressional committees have been challenging the heretofore unchallengeable: the medical establishment and its aura of sacrosanctity."

Owen McNamara, *Providence Journal*

"*White Coat, Clenched Fist* is a useful presentation of one side of the metamorphosis of the 1960s campus radicalism into experiments and programs of the 1970s. But its greater relevance lies in what it can tell us about the obstacles to thoroughgoing change to our system of medical care."

Jerry Avorn, *Working Papers*

"Mullan's narrative recalls the progression that so many people went through in the 1960s and early 1970s: from liberal support of the civil rights movement to opposition of the War in Vietnam to an all embracing radical critique of American society. . . . His discussion of the politics of health as he and his fellow medical students and doctors encountered it not only illuminates a fascinating, little understood period of our recent history but also gives life to what has become an essentially statistical debate over proposals for a national health plan."

Ron Dorfman, *Chicago Magazine*

CONVERSATIONS IN MEDICINE AND SOCIETY

The Conversations in Medicine and Society series publishes innovative, accessible, and provocative books on a range of topics related to health, society, culture, and policy in modern America (1900 to the present). Current and upcoming titles focus on the historical, social, and cultural dimensions of health and sickness, public policy, medical professionalization, and subjective experiences of illness.

Series Editors
Howard Markel and Alexandra Minna Stern,
University of Michigan

Formative Years: Children's Health in the United States, 1800–2000
edited by Alexandra Minna Stern and Howard Markel

The DNA Mystique: The Gene as Cultural Icon
by Dorothy Nelkin and M. Susan Lindee

Universal Coverage: The Elusive Quest for National Health Insurance
by Rick Mayes

*The Midnight Meal and Other Essays
About Doctors, Patients, and Medicine*
by Jerome Lowenstein

*Deadly Dust: Silicosis and the On-Going Struggle
to Protect Workers' Health*
by David Rosner and Gerald Markowitz

Inside/Outside: A Physician's Journey with Breast Cancer
by Janet R. Gilsdorf

*White Coat, Clenched Fist:
The Political Education of an American Physician*
by Fitzhugh Mullan

White Coat, Clenched Fist

THE POLITICAL EDUCATION OF AN AMERICAN PHYSICIAN

Fitzhugh Mullan, M.D.

THE UNIVERSITY OF MICHIGAN PRESS
Ann Arbor

Library of Congress Cataloging-in-Publication Data

Mullan, Fitzhugh.
    White coat, clenched fist : the political education of an American
physician / Fitzhugh Mullan.
        p. ; cm. — (Conversations in medicine and society)
    Includes bibliographical references and index.
    ISBN-13: 978-0-472-03197-9 (alk. paper)
    ISBN-10: 0-472-03197-X (alk. paper)
    1. Physicians—United States—Biography. 2. Medical education—
United States. 3. Medical care—United States. I. Title. II. Series.

[DNLM: 1. Education, Medical—United States—Personal Narratives.
2. Physicians—United States—Personal Narratives. WZ 100 M955w 2006]

R154.M856A33   2006
610.92—dc22
    [B]   2006051058

To new generations of healers:
question, challenge, change

Certain of the persons mentioned in this book are referred to by fictional names in order to insure that their identities remain concealed.

Foreword

Howard Markel, M.D., Ph.D., and Alexandra Minna Stern, Ph.D.

At a time in which our health care system is often criticized for privileging profits over people, the reissue of Fitzhugh Mullan's *White Coat, Clenched Fist* seems particularly apt. Written over thirty years ago as a kind of immediate memoir, *White Coat, Clenched Fist* chronicled how direct involvement in the civil rights movement shaped Mullan's ideas and approaches to doctoring in America. As Dr. Mullan explains in his new preface, when he wrote *White Coat, Clenched Fist* in the mid-1970s, he infused the memoir with the optimism he felt at the time. Namely, that Americans had committed to the health of the poor and underprivileged with Medicare and Medicaid, supported the development of many community-based health programs, and that the demographic profile of physicians was changing and becoming more inclusive of women and minorities.

Fast-forward to 2006 and Mullan's optimism has been wrenchingly replaced by outrage and dismay. Instead of the fulfillment of the promise of 1960s health care reform, the last several decades have witnessed the relentless privatization and corporatization of health care, whether in the form of exorbitant insurance premiums, expensive technological advances, or unaffordable medications. We agree with Mullan that these dramatic changes make his memoir even more relevant and illuminating today. Indeed, *White Coat, Clenched Fist* has itself become a historical document that can transport us to another—not too distant—era in American society. As historians of medicine, we believe that it is important for medical students and health care professionals today to have access to Mullan's personal journey of radicalization and professionalization. Thus, we are delighted that, after decades of being out of print, this book is available to the public.

Even as *White Coat, Clenched Fist* captures a particular moment, it should be noted that it was an early stepping-stone for Mullan's impressive career as a public intellectual; he subsequently penned many publications, ranging from a cancer memoir to a book celebrating the lives of everyday heroes, primary care physicians. Moreover, through endeavors such as the editorship of the "Narrative Matters" column in the policy journal *Health Affairs* Dr. Mullan has sought to provide a venue for health care workers who believe the pen, or in our day the computer keyboard, serves as an important vehicle to express personal experience of medicine, health, and healing.

To this day, Dr. Mullan continues to speak for an articulate minority of physicians who have dedicated their careers to treating the country's most vulnerable citizens. In many respects, he embodies the title of our series, Conversations in Medicine and Society, as he has initiated many important conversations about the state of the American health care system—its physicians, nurses, and patients. Luckily for us, Mullan insists that this conversation, even if noisy and difficult at times, continue.

Preface:
The Clenched Fist Revisited

It is forty-plus years since a personal awakening that took place in a community called Second Pilgrims' Rest in Holmes County, Mississippi. I was a twenty-three-year-old, first-year medical student unhappy with my chosen profession, disturbed about the race divide in America, and desperately eager to find a way of life that made sense to me. What I encountered in Mississippi that summer—poverty, hope, racism, bravery, friendship, and mission—provide a spiritual and vocational gyroscope for the rest of my life. *White Coat, Clenched Fist: The Political Education of an American Physician* is a chronicle of that Mississippi summer and the decade that followed of political activism, educational reform, and social confrontation. It was the decade of the civil rights movement, the Vietnam War, and Watergate. It was a decade of intense political engagement by people from all walks of life, including young physicians who challenged the traditional role of medicine in American life.

When I wrote *White Coat* it was with the strong urge to tell all, to document what I had seen and lived through, to pass on what I had learned—the wisdom and insights as well as the failures and shortcomings to which I had been a party. I wanted to instruct, exhort, warn, and encourage others who shared my concerns. *White Coat* was to be a travelers' guide to radicalism in medicine and reform in medical education. I wanted others to travel the route I had taken, but I wanted them to have the benefit of my experiences.

The intersection between radical politics and American medicine does not occupy a large space. Although *White Coat* was treated with favorable reviews and I spent some time on talk shows around the country, the book sold a modest number of copies, never had a paperback printing, and was out of print within several years. It turns out, however, that the intersection between radical politics and American medicine is an enduring one. Some number of students from every generation is concerned about inequities in medicine, and a substantial group of practitioners is devoted to reform strategies. *White Coat* has lived on in the libraries of these physicians and others committed to basic change in U.S. health care. To my surprise and gratification, the book seems to have served well as a travelogue for medical reformers.

At its current age it is also history. The issues, events, and people are now part of our national legacy. They have a richer and fuller context that allows them to be examined with the objectivity of hindsight. The historical travelogue has a lot to say about the past and also about the present. It is in that spirit that I believe the University of Michigan Press has decided to reissue *White Coat, Clenched Fist* and that I offer the following thoughts about the "clenched fist" revisited.

Taking Stock

The sixties were a watershed for this country. It was the time of the civil rights movement, the women's movement, and the antiwar movement, all of which were vital elements of our national life and of my life then—with reverberations to the present. It was a time of objection and a time of reform, and while the expression of those sentiments was not always neatly packaged or clearly articulated, the message was strong and consistent: the complacent, bland, smug, post–World War II America of the 1950s was chock full of double standards, hypocrisy, and racism. Segregation was embedded in custom and law. Half of society (women) was consigned to presumptive secondary status and limited opportunities. The escalating war in Vietnam seemed a bloody exercise in the export of these hypocritical values and a spectacular waste of life on both sides.

The world of medicine that I discovered in medical school was riddled with similar inequities. One in ten students in my medical school class was a woman. One in seventy-two was black—and he came from Nigeria. The main functions of the Student American Medical Association (SAMA) on campus was social, and the American Medical Association was engaged in a last ditch effort to prevent the enactment of Medicare to provide health insurance for the nation's elderly. A student did not have to arrive in medicine as a radical to be troubled by the moral posture of the profession in the 1960s.

My experiences in Mississippi started my journey as an activist—a journey whose next decade is detailed in *White Coat, Clenched Fist.*

For me, as for others, that activism was both political and cultural. In medicine we challenged medical schools on admissions and curriculum, hospitals on public accountability, the military on the doctor draft, and our colleagues in medicine on their values and priorities. The cultural confrontation in medicine was less dramatic than in the society as a whole. There never was a medical Woodstock or the clinical equivalent of bra burning. Beards did become more prominent, students were included in many more medical school committees, residency night coverage was made less onerous, and eventually the numbers of women entering medicine increased dramatically. From the trivial to the critical, the sixties triggered a slow but significant culture change in medicine.

By the time I wrote *White Coat,* the sixties were over literally and figuratively. The ubiquitous protests of earlier years had subsided, the war in Vietnam had ended, the Voting Rights Act was on the books, and formalized segregation was defeated. When *White Coat* was published in 1976, there was reason to look at the previous decade with a sense of accomplishment and toward the future with a sense of promise. Segregation had been ended, the war was over, opportunities for women were expanding rapidly. In medicine, Medicare and Medicaid were up and functioning, as were the newly enacted Community Health Center program and the National Health Service Corps. Community medicine departments existed in most medical schools, and women and blacks were being admitted in record numbers. Whatever else the sixties had been, in medicine they seemed to have delivered a victory for fairness. It was true that many Americans still lacked health insurance, but "national health insurance" was on the public agenda, discussed by none less than Presidents Nixon and Carter, and surely was only a legislative session or two away. Although medical school was still the preserve of the wealthy, new affirmative action programs and government scholarships promised to bring greater democracy and equity to medical education in the near future. In 1976 a medical activist had reason to feel satisfaction with the past and hope for the future.

Course Change

The election of Ronald Reagan to the presidency in 1980 stunned me. I could not believe that the majority of the country bought the conservative platitudes of a lightweight movie actor. Who were these people? Hadn't Barry Goldwater been repudiated in 1964? Didn't the world of oil crises, rising nationalism, and mammoth wealth disparities call for more sophisticated political leadership than a rosy-cheeked man calling for "morning in America"?

My reaction to the Reagan election proved, in retrospect, to be a commentary on me and my political presumptions. Large parts of America had remained staunchly conservative, comfortably isolationist, and fiercely individualistic. This reality, combined with artful constituency building by neoconservatives, solidified the new conservatism. The strategic creation of right-wing think tanks in Washington, the rapid and highly politicized cultivation of fundamentalist instincts led by the religious right, the insertion of abortion politics as a schismatic and diversionary bomblet into every aspect of political discourse, and the rise of the radio talk show demagogues for the purpose of feeding all of the above rank as a monumental hijacking of the U.S. political process. The result of these innovations has been activist conservative presidencies for five of the last seven terms.

My incredulity at the Reagan election and the subsequent Republican victories in multiple national elections is a commentary on the simplicity of my thinking in 1980. Yes, the sixties had made America a more progressive country with increasing attention to liberal values and equality in the distribution of resources. This was certainly true of the multiple legislative innovations in the health sector. What I missed entirely was the residual hardcore individualism of many Americans— a well-established characteristic of this nation from de Tocqueville on and one that was (and is) a powerful receptor site for conservative exhortations. We may believe in being our brother's keeper between ten and one o'clock on Sunday mornings, but we're not so clear about it the rest of the week. Ronald Reagan and his strategists understood this.

As young people in medicine, we monumentally misjudged the battles of the future. We thought that the American Medical Association and the self-interested domination of health policy by doctors were to be the principal antagonists of the future. In the thirty years since *White Coat* was published, the AMA has dwindled in influence due in part to its own stumbling and in part to the changing political landscape for which it likewise was ill prepared. Insurance companies, with their grip on individual health benefits; drug companies, with their direct-to-the-individual appeal (for both longer life and greater sexual fulfillment); and medical equipment manufacturers, pushing items such as individual implantable cardioverter defibrillators, are the most powerful forces in our chaotic, expensive, and ongoing national struggle over health care access, costs, and quality. In health, as elsewhere in public life these days, collective values have a bad name. Communitarian principles are in retreat. Medicaid is a target for cutbacks. The Community Health Center program, enacted as part of the War on Poverty in 1965 as a stopgap for communities that had no health services, is now supported, ironically, as a permanent "safety net program"— part of the have and have-not, upstairs/downstairs rationale of conservative thinking. "The Ownership Society" is the mantra of conservative thinking and the Bush administration. Virtually any legislative proposal aimed at making the system more equitable or affordable has to genuflect to "market solutions."

Prior to 1970, a nonprofit presumption held sway in medicine. Although physicians were certainly well paid and many firms such as drug companies made profits from medical products, medicine's business ethic was minimally commercial and nonprofit oriented. Doctors did not advertise. Hospitals were tax-exempt not-for-profit community institutions. Much of American philanthropy was devoted to supporting the medical sector, and patients were not the subject of commercial appeals by business interests.

The rise of for-profit hospitals in the 1970s signaled the breaching of the levees for medical commercialism. Numerous business interests followed the groundbreaking medical commercialism of firms such as the Hospital Corporation of America and National Medical Enterprises. For-profit health insurance companies quickly replaced the nonprofit Blue Cross and Blue Shield organizations as predominant health insurance carriers in America. The Blues themselves began to morph into for-profit entities. The basic premise of insurance is shared risk— we are all in this together. This often means that the healthy contribute to financing care for the sick with the certain expectation that one day they too will be sick. The young help out with the old, the generally healthy with the unexpectedly sick, and so on. Commercial insurance, however, requires profits. To the standard employer-based health plans and government-sponsored Medicare and Medicaid programs were added an increasing array of managed care plans that featured endless ways of dividing patients and benefits. Inexorably, plans pitched to younger or healthier groups cost less, appealed to the target population, and succeeded financially. Each disaggregation of risk that occurred, however, meant that older, sicker, and often poorer patients would have to pay more, rely on the government, or go without insurance.

By the 1990s, a blizzard of managed-care schemes mixing insurance, service delivery, and sometimes physician gatekeepers emerged as alternatives to traditional insurance. Physicians began to advertise. Patients became "customers." The FDA relaxed previous prohibitions against direct-to-consumer advertising, resulting in relentless sales pitches to the public. Political leaders riding the tide of commercialism countenanced the growth of an ever more expensive health care system that has carried with it many of the disparities that the reforms of the sixties and seventies were on a trajectory to reduce or eliminate. Nothing approaching national health insurance has passed Congress. The bold effort of the Clinton administration to reform the system as a whole ended as a massive political debacle. The number of uninsured in the country is high and growing. We spend 50 percent more per capita on health care in the United States than the next most munificent nation (Norway) yet have health outcomes in many areas that place us well down in the ranks of industrialized nations. We have no national physician training policy despite spending $8 billion a year subsidizing hospitals to produce the most heavily specialized physician workforce in the world. We have recently doubled the budget of the NIH, renewing our commitment to medical innovation while holding constant the tiny budget of the program responsible for medical quality and evaluation (the Agency for Healthcare Research and Quality). Today we spend one dollar on evaluation for every hundred we invest in innovation. Without stated purpose but with disturbingly steady step we have put in place policies that create new technology, stimulate expenditures, deprecate planning, ignore evaluation, and promote "markets" to serve those with money or entitlements.

Boutique or concierge medicine is, perhaps, the high temple of the new individualist/market mentality in medical care. Numbers of physicians in private practice who dislike the complexities of modern practice, the uncertainties of the insurance system, and what they feel is the high volume of patients for whom they are accountable have seceded from the system. These physicians close their practices and reopen them to a much smaller, wealthier clientele. They accept insurance generally but, in addition, require a retainer of some thousands of dollars a year from each patient. For the retainer in addition to their fees, they promise their patients longer office visits, rapid responsiveness, and a general increase in TLC. Patients who can afford this arrangement often think it is a terrific idea for them personally. One does not have to contemplate this scenario for long to appreciate the problems that boutique medicine portends for the system as a whole. The physicians choosing this route practice only with wealthy patients and have renounced a substantial number of the people for whom they had previously cared. The system is the worse for their decision. Boutique medicine reverts to the notion of the physician as shopkeeper—a shop established for the privileged few who can afford the amenities provided in a doting way by the medical shopkeeper. One cannot escape the conclusion that Marie Antoinette would have understood and approved such a system.

The Twenty-first Century

The Old World was simpler. In the sixties, the adversary was clear. It was the unfairness, hypocrisy, and self-satisfaction of a system symbolized by the AMA—medicine's good old boys' club. Male, white, rich, blind to the inequities in America, and successful over and over again in opposing change, the AMA was the embodiment of the failed potential of medicine in the United States as we saw it then.

Cuba was our hero. The Cuban Revolution was the symbol of socialism and of the politically articulated principles of people uniting to throw off repression and build new societies. Che even more than Fidel symbolized a worldwide movement that fought for the poor, reached out to previously colonized people, promoted the rights of women and minorities, and was undaunted by the West's capitalism. We were not Communists, but the existence of the international socialist movement inspired us and represented a counterbalance to the stolid, self-interested dominance of conservative politics that was our reality and that the AMA represented so mightily in medicine.

Today the world is different. The AMA's earlier role as the voice of the medical profession is challenged daily by a variety of other medical organizations and dozens of potent nonphysician interest groups baying at the Congress and the public. While Fidel soldiers on in Cuba, the Soviet bloc is gone. So, too, is the international movement it fostered, which underscored the rights and needs of the poor and contested the market precepts of capitalism.

The goals and the heroes of the sixties are gone, leaving a world that is politically much more complicated. As medical student activists of the sixties have grown and aged, we have chosen a variety of routes to express our political commitments. Many have worked in government, public health, and management activities, instinctively trying to steer the health care system in principled directions. Some have chosen specific areas in which to labor such as prison health, international health, child health, and medical journalism. Many continue to work with activist movements such as Physicians for Social Responsibility, Physicians for Human Rights, and Physicians for a National Health Program. This last effort enlists physicians in a national campaign for a single-payer system and comes as close as anything to an organizational home for the medical activist sentiments of the 1960s.

A brief but powerful rallying point for physicians eager to reform the system was the election of Bill Clinton as president and his two-year effort to reconstitute the U.S. health care system. The years 1992 to 1994 provided opportunities for many health activists who had their roots in the sixties to work in the Old Executive Office Building adjacent to the White House and draft legislative proposals for everything from Indian health to health informatics. Unfortunately the reform campaign failed due to poor political management and the effective opposition of conservatives and commercial interests. This failure dealt a blow to the idea of civic reform in the health system that reverberates yet today.

Throughout the latter part of the twentieth century, the principal medical student organization in the country has remained faithful to the principles established by the activists of the sixties. The Student Health Organization (SHO) lived a meteoric life in the 1960s. The SHO (whose history is chronicled in *White Coat*) burst onto the medical school scene in 1965 as a symbol of and vehicle for student activism and curriculum reform. The entrenched student group at the time, the Student American Medical Association (SAMA), was an organization that generally oversaw microscope exchanges and campus dances. It had no political agenda, at least none that challenged the reigning order in medical education and practice. One of the common themes of the Student Health Organization was its objection to the abdication of student politics by SAMA. From its start SHO was dedicated to engaging students in the issues of the time and to doing so with the sense of social conscience— a time-honored student role. During the late 1960s, the leadership of SAMA was successively affronted, threatened, and finally recruited by the strategies and successes of the Student Health Organization. The strategies included curriculum reform, community service projects, and the generation of external funding. The SHO was successful in securing substantial government and private foundation support.

Lacking a formal national structure, often organized around charismatic individuals, and increasingly antiwar in focus, the SHO slowly fell apart in the late 1960s. Its antiwar stance effectively terminated government support, and foundations were skeptical of funding the poorly organized remnants of the earlier movement. On the other hand,

SAMA had a formalized and stable national structure that provided for an orderly turnover in national leadership each year, as well as an apparatus of trustees and committees that involved most of the country's medical schools. SAMA and its leaders quickly adopted programs that included community service, curriculum reform, and, ultimately, external funding very much in the spirit of the Student Health Organization.

In recognition of its new activism and in the desire to set a distance between itself and the American Medical Association, SAMA changed its name in 1972 to the American Medical Student Association (AMSA) and, to a large degree, has continued the principles of medical student activism ever since. Year after year AMSA has attracted students to its leadership ranks who are interested in social change and medical reform. It has sponsored numerous programs of community engagement with funds from government agencies such as the National Health Service Corps and the Community Health Center program. AMSA publications and annual meetings have tended to feature topics and speakers challenging the medical status quo. Many AMSA officers from earlier years have gone on to important leadership positions in government, medical education, and medical reform initiatives. Through the changing world of medical politics over its thirty years, AMSA has remained remarkably constant in its invocation of the need for change and the importance of students as bearers of that message.

Personal Journey

Despite my personal frustrations with the evolution of medicine in America since *White Coat* was first published, my life in medicine has been fascinating and fulfilling. In fact, what might be called the equity doldrums of American medicine over the last thirty years have provided endless employment opportunities for those of us with a bent for medical reform. Following three years in New Mexico as a National Health Service Corps physician, I returned to Washington, where I became director of the NHSC during the Carter administration. I spent the following years (twenty-three in all) as a commissioned officer in the U.S. Public Health Service, spending time at the NIH, working on the staff of Surgeon General Koop, serving as Secretary of Health and Environment for the state of New Mexico, and running the Federal Bureau of Health Professions during the first Clinton administration. Public service and political management are important roles for activists and reformers. But the possibilities of public management are largely defined by national politics—a politics that has tended to move away from the ideal of health equity rather than toward it. The promise of the Clinton health care reform effort followed by its collapse prompted me to leave government and return to more primary medical pursuits. I did this not in the spirit that government is a failure or that reformers shouldn't work in government. To the contrary, work in the public sector is essential to good government and to improved health care in America. Rather, I was ready to tackle reform from a different angle.

Today, thirty years after the publication of *White Coat,* I am a teacher at the George Washington University. I conduct policy research on global health workforce issues; I practice pediatrics at a community health center in Washington, DC; and I continue to write. But teaching health policy and pediatrics to medical and public health students is my core mission. It is not hard to find students who share the *White Coat* view of the unfulfilled agenda of U.S. medicine. Many are activist by inclination and arrive at school enthusiastic about their chosen careers but disturbed by the blatant waste and unfairness in our nation's health care system. Each of these students is a potential agent of change, a latter-day sixties activist, a new healer destined to challenge and improve the system.

It is to them, their colleagues elsewhere in the country, and those who follow them as students of the health sciences that I dedicate the reissued *White Coat, Clenched Fist.* Health equity remains the goal. The sixties are their legacy. I offer them *White Coat* and its glimpse of the past to help them chart their future courses.

Washington, DC
June, 2006

Contents

Introduction

When I left Lincoln Hospital in 1972 I felt that I had a story to tell. The tale was a specific one—the history of a New York municipal hospital, born of nineteenth-century charity, steeped in evolving racism, woefully antiquated in the present era of organ transplants and cataract removals. The story of Lincoln appealed to me because I thought it was important history; it told us something about the past and a great deal about the present.

As I began to write, the work began to change. My earliest critics all proved more interested in how I got to Lincoln (where I worked for two tumultuous years) and what happened while I was there than they were in the blow-by-blow history of the institution itself. They wanted to know what a young white physician with firm middle-class roots was doing in a dilapidated, strife-torn, black and Puerto Rican hospital in the South Bronx. So, gradually, the book became my own story, the story of a young American growing up in medicine.

My family is deeply rooted in medicine. My father's father hoped to become a naval officer like his father. He failed in his effort to gain admission to the United States Naval Academy at Annapolis and so entered medicine, graduating from the University of Maryland Medical School in 1905. He spent his life in the United States Public Health Service working largely in the area of immigration. For many years he was stationed at Ellis Island in New York harbor. I have often wondered what percentage of America passed under his examining hands. My father did go to the Naval Academy but then turned to medicine, graduating from Cornell University Medical School in 1939. He has practiced psychiatry and group psychotherapy for thirty years. I think that the particular radicalism and nonconformity of his practice have been a consistent positive influence on me.

My medical experience has been wholly different from that of my father or grandfather. Clearly our times, which are different from theirs, have influenced me. More than that, though, I have approached medicine in a consistently less accepting way than they did. Perhaps it is out of some need to differentiate myself from them. Perhaps it is because the necessity for change in medicine is ever so much more obvious today than it was thirty or sixty years ago. But the fact is that I have never felt comfortable with medicine as it is taught, organized, or practiced in the United States.

To some degree I am sure that that discomfort is of my own genesis. To some degree it is not. Like all cultural expressions, American medicine has a style, a personality and a politics; the politics, in particular, are far more pronounced than the aloof white coat might suggest. Moreover, medicine in the United States has generally received less scrutiny and criticism than other elements of the body social—the school system and the courts, for instance. Most people have strong opinions about "their" doctors but have less informed and less decisive comments about the practice and organization of medicine as a whole. The technological aspects of medicine as well as its priestly overtones have tended to prevent people from exacting as rigorous a criticism of medical practice as they might. In any event, American medicine is not often examined from a political perspective. Who goes into medicine and why? What happens to them when they do? What are they taught that is not strictly scientific and what do they come to expect? What happens to them after they leave medical school and begin to practice their newly acquired skills? And what does this mean for the patients of America—*all* of us?

As I began to record my own experiences in medical school, internship, and residency, I found that the persistent theme was my own awakening to the nonmedical and nonscientific forces that were shaping my education. Human, sometimes disturbing, frequently powerful, these forces were not the items that medical educators usually write about when characterizing the academic experience. Moreover, most of them were not the kind of things that the public envisions their doctors spending time and energy learning. But they were real, time-consuming, and, for better or for worse, character-forming. To a large extent, these were the forces that shape the personality of American medicine. Put simply, they were the politics of an education in medicine in the present epoch.

So *White Coat, Clenched Fist* became the story of my political education as a physician. In fairness, I was not a passive observer in that process, and the book as it has emerged is hardly a dispassionate account of health care in America. But that was never my intent. The book is my story; yet it is not that alone. It is the experience of a group and, to an extent, a generation of young people in medicine who since the mid-1960s have consistently questioned the structure of American medicine. Collectively we have learned medicine and learned about medicine, and collectively we have labored to change it. The story remains to be completed but that which is already history can teach us a good deal. It is in that spirit that I write.

Garrett Park, Maryland
March, 1976

White Coat, Clenched Fist

1

Mississippi Nightwatch

"Cat. You stay awake. D'you hear? Fall asleep and they'll kill you." All I could see of Cat was a red, glowing cigarette ash. "I hear you, Mr. Sills. I won't sleep. I promise." I couldn't see Mr. Sills at all. "Promise, nothing. If you care about your hide you'll keep your eyes open and your ears sharp. It's your only hope."

Cat, Mr. Sills, and I sat in the dark in front of a dilapidated country church in Holmes County, Mississippi. Cat and Mr. Sills were local black farmers and members of the church. I was a medical student from Chicago who had come to Mississippi as a civil rights worker. The year was 1965.

"They tried to burn this church down once and if they come back they'll be meaner than before. You know what they'll do if they find you here?"

"What, Mr. Sills?"

"They'll shoot you first, probably before you wake up 'cause I've seen how you sleep. Then they'll pour gasoline all over your body and the church and light it up. They'll say you was a no-good-civil-rights-nigger and got burned up messing with your own church."

"I won't fall asleep. Really I won't, Mr. Sills."

The three of us sat in the dark holding shotguns on our laps. Cat smoked his cigarettes and Mr. Sills sipped water from a canteen. The hours passed slowly. The previous week someone had tried to fire-bomb the building, leaving an ugly black scar on one wall. The church hosted the weekly meeting of the Freedom Democratic party, the local civil rights organization, and thus became a target for a group of young whites from a nearby town. The black community had decided to defend their church rather than see it destroyed. So we took turns spending our nights sitting in the dark listening to the sounds of the Mississippi countryside, fingering our guns, and hoping nobody would come up the road.

I spent many hours at the church thinking back over my first year of medical school, which had ended only two months before. The microscopes and dog dissections, the lectures and labs seemed far distant. I could remember the grueling, unpleasant year in detail and yet in many ways it seemed never to have happened. It had been obliterated, overwhelmed by the experience in Mississippi.

The Civil Rights Movement was so much more real, so much more compelling. The people with whom I lived and worked were locked in a battle to remake their lives and to destroy the system of racism that permeated their world. The struggle was in earnest, one side prepared to take life and the other willing to give it to win. There was a sense of history, of brotherhood, and of fear in much of what we did. By contrast medical school was contrived and dull. The first year had passed as a long, drab rehearsal—a rehearsal for a time when we would deal with real people and real problems. We practiced for the day when we would be physicians. We learned to memorize; we stockpiled information; we pulled apart a human corpse and we sacrificed a dozen dogs, mechanically reproducing physiological principles spelled out in our texts. But we did nothing real. Where labs had been tedious and stultifying, the South proved combustible. Where school demanded competitiveness and bred alienation, the Civil Rights Movement offered the kinship and warmth of common struggle. I suffered through the first year of medicine because it was an investment for the future. I guarded the church because I believed in it.

"Cat," called Mr. Sills softly. There was no answer. "Cat," he called again louder. Still no answer. "Damn kid. I knew it was no use having him out here. Gone to sleep, just like I said." I could see Cat's slumped form vaguely outlined against the wall of the church. I got up to wake him, but Mr. Sills stopped me. "No use. He'll just doze off again. I know him. Let him sleep."

We were quiet for a while and then Mr. Sills started to talk. "Fifty-two years I've lived in this country. All my fifty-two years. This is the first time anything like this has ever happened and it's about time. I been chopping cotton and picking cotton almost fifty years and what do I have to show for it? Five acres of land, a house that's a shack and a '56 Chevy pickup. Now that isn't too bad in some ways, but it's not much to show for all those years of work. It keeps me and the wife alive but really it isn't much. This here civil rights is going to make things a lot better. At least for my grandkids. That's why we got to keep this church in one piece."

Mr. Sills's reasons were like those of the other men who spent their nights standing watch and like those of the many black families who attended the Freedom Democratic party meeting at the church every Wednesday night. They understood clearly the racism they suffered under and they sensed that life would be better without it. In song and in prayer their struggle was spiritual, yet at heart the Movement was pragmatic. In Holmes County in 1965 blacks received three dollars for a full day in the fields; they were severely limited as to how many acres of their own land they could plant in cotton (the money crop); very few could vote; and none attended "white" schools. Mr. Sills knew that changing these conditions would change his life; for that he joined the Civil Rights Movement.

At least on the surface my reasons for guarding the church were quite different. White, raised in the North, the son of well-to-do parents, I had never suffered from racism. My life was neither harassed nor limited by racial politics. Raised in New York City, educated in private schools, I grew up in relative racial seclusion. My principal black acquaintances were an occasional, carefully chosen, scholarship schoolmate, the cleaning lady, the doorman. At thirteen I left home for a New England boarding school where the words "nigger" and "coon" as well as "kike" and "jewboy" were very popular. The traditionalist school educated no blacks and only a few Jews, yet many students derived pleasure or status from the repeated use of racial epithets. Racial consciousness and racism were part of my youth even if interracial exposure was not.

When I entered Harvard College in 1960 my major concerns were passing (something I was not at all sure I could do) and figuring out what I wanted to do with my life. I was glad to find the racism (I called it "prejudice") I had seen in boarding school less conspicuous in the cosmopolitan Cambridge surroundings. Yet the early 1960s were not an easy time to remain apolitical at Harvard. It was the epoch of the New Frontier which appeared to be made for the youthful energies of me and my classmates. McGeorge Bundy, Arthur Schlesinger, and Ted Sorensen were all taken from our classrooms to serve in Washington. The Peace Corps and the War on Poverty seemed designed for us. We hobnobbed with the sons and daughters of Administration leaders who were in abundance in Cambridge. John Kennedy himself was on the Board of Overseers of Harvard and, while still president-elect, visited the campus. Many planned careers in politics or public service. Washington seemed but a year or two away and we assumed that the youthful, vibrant New Frontier would be there to take us in and put us to work. We sensed an intimacy with power that, real or not, gave rise to excitement and optimism. More important perhaps, the power seemed to us compassionate, imaginative, and strong.

But it was not just Administration and establishment politics that appealed to me. Although I perceived little difference at the time, the early sixties saw the birth of the politics of protest. Civil rights and peace were coming issues. I read enthusiastically about sit-ins and Freedom Rides, and Harvard students formed a campus organization to send money and people South to support the nascent Civil Rights Movement. In 1961 I marched in the streets for the first time under the banner of SANE (the Society for the Abolition of Nuclear Explosions) and, in 1962, worked hard for a peace candidate for the U.S. Senate, Harvard professor H. Stuart Hughes. Hughes campaigned well but a week before the election the Cuban missile crisis broke and he was badly beaten by another political newcomer who took a harder line on weapons, Ted Kennedy.

"Trouble with defending yourself in this country," said Mr. Sills after a long silence, "is that it ain't easy. First a person's got to make up his mind that he's tired of taking crap and that he's ready to fight. That's tough to do—but that's the easy part."

"What do you mean?" I asked.

"Well it ain't easy to decide to stand up to some of these white folk around here. Specially after you ain't done it for so long. It's hard to join the Civil Rights. But once you have, it gets tough. If we got to shoot a man—a white man—to defend this church, things'll get pretty hot for us. You can't imagine the law laying off us around here even if it was self-defense and the man was trespassing. No sir. They'd string us up just like we shot a man while we were trying to burn down *his* church. They won't let us defend ourselves if we want to."

"So why are we out here at all?" I queried.

"If we shoot, we take to the woods. There's no way they'll find us out there. Those are our woods. We'll teach them a lesson, but we don't need to be heroes. They can't string us up if they don't know who we are."

I didn't like Mr. Sills's idea much. The woods weren't *my* woods and I couldn't see myself playing guerrilla, even for a short time. Moreover, I had grown up with a belief in the law. If a man wanted to defend his church against someone who tried to burn it down, he shouldn't have to run and hide. Yet Mr. Sills knew Mississippi and I had to respect his instincts. Even I had trouble envisioning a local jury acquitting a black for shooting a white regardless of the circumstances. If Mr. Sills ran, I resolved, I would run too and do my best to keep up with him.

After a time I fell to thinking about school again. It was during my senior year at Harvard that I began to seriously consider getting involved in the Civil Rights Movement. An increased knowledge of segregation and the inequities that resulted from it angered me. More than that, I found the spirit of change and redress that surrounded the Movement compelling. Somewhat simplistically it seemed to me that the work of our generation was to end segregation once and for all. At base, the Civil Rights Movement appealed to me for reasons I find hard to articulate. It seemed right, it was timely, and I wanted to be part of it. The year 1964 produced "Freedom Summer," the first large-scale assault of northern youth on southern racism. The appeal went out to students across the country to go South, sponsored by the Student Non-violent Coordinating Committee (SNCC) and the Council of Federated Organizations (COFO). Hundreds went, including two close friends of mine, but I did not. I had applied to medical school and in order to be admitted in the fall I had to study embryology.

I had thought for a number of years about becoming a physician. Medicine appealed to me because it was a practical art that would allow me to work closely with people. I recognized that the romance of my political and social thinking needed to be matched by some tangible skill to make it useful. The practice of medicine seemed to offer an intimacy with people and their problems that would allow me to exercise my personal principles in a useful way. Yet I found the premedical competition disheartening and I disliked science courses and took as few as possible. Moreover, the image of the American physician always disturbed me. I could not see myself as a member of the American Medical Association. I feared the white-coat socialization process that awaited me. Was I to become a booster of the country club, plump, Goldwaterite, the darling of stock brokers and life insurance salesmen? I doubted it, but prospects looked bleak, judging by the relatively few doctors who seemed to escape that fate. Certainly afternoons and evenings consumed by science labs—with more to come in medical school—promised to steal one's youth and breed some kind of greed for reparations.

In the end, I went to medical school for extremely practical and, really, conservative reasons—the same reasons, more or less, for which my classmates went. Medicine could be counted on. It was a defined, needed, remunerative career. "I want to write an epic poem. I want to write a poem they'll remember me for," a classmate told me on the way to an anatomy lab. "I want to write it now. But it didn't happen to me yesterday—nor this morning. So I'm going to this crappy lab this afternoon and I suppose I'll keep going." He's a neurologist now.

The summer of 1964 was a difficult time for me, confronted squarely as I was by my ambivalence about medicine. While hundreds of young Americans went South to try to change history I busied myself with yolk sacs and pig fetuses. I studied the significance of the neural crest while the nation recoiled at the murders of three civil rights workers in Philadelphia, Mississippi. Embryology seemed particularly trivial and irrelevant in the face of Freedom Summer but it proved to be only a warm-up for what was to come in the fall. In September I began medical school at the University of Chicago. Anatomy, biochemistry, and physiology were the grist of the first year—a decision made by medical educators around the turn of the century and carried out doggedly by medical schools ever since. Our basic curriculum included only one contact that could in any way be construed as interchange with a patient—and that was our anatomy cadaver. In an effort to cope with our own repugnance at the dissection of the human body and, perhaps, with the hope of dignifying our one patient contact, we named our corpse "Granny." She yielded her secrets to our scalpels sinew by sinew as the year passed.

After the initial shock of anatomy lab, I accustomed myself to the daily visit with our elderly lady friend, but I had difficulty accepting the need to memorize the position of every nerve, vein, tendon, muscle, joint, and bone in her withered body. Anatomy was an assault on me—me, the young person, the history major, the pre-med who disliked blood and strong odors and was awed by death. Anatomy was an attack on my mind—an average, college-educated, twenty-two-year-old mind that enjoyed reading, speculating, pondering, and fantasizing. Making me lab partners with a corpse whose every innard I was supposed to probe was a toughening and, I do not doubt, a mind-altering experience. I never could bring myself to do it, but many zealous classmates ate lunch on their cadavers while dissecting. Then, too, anatomy was an intellectual hurdle. We were responsible for knowing literally every element of the body and its relation to every other element—tens of thousands of separate pieces of knowledge—

a reservoir of information equivalent to learning a foreign language with a large vocabulary. The catch was that this was a language we would never use. The amount of anatomy actually needed in the day-to-day practice of medicine could be found in the equivalent of a Berlitz pocket dictionary.

Our examinations reflected the blind, anti-intellectual quality of our work. We all assembled outside the door of the anatomy lab at the appointed time. The spirit of the occasion reminded me of waiting outside the living-room door on Christmas morning—I knew I would recognize the place but it would be rearranged and full of surprises. Our professor, a portly South African who chain-smoked cigars (to kill the odor, we speculated), never failed us. The door opened and we bustled in and took up positions in front of a cadaver, any cadaver. At the signal we were to study the organ, nerve, or vessel marked with a colored pin. We had precisely sixty seconds to make the identification, at the end of which a wind-up kitchen timer would sound in our hall of science and we would move on to the next pinned cadaver and start our labors again. After we had been the whole circuit we had three free minutes during which we could look at whatever we liked. Pandemonium reigned. Then the exam was over and, supposedly, we were one small step closer to being doctors of medicine, physicians to the human being.

What was anatomy all about? This was a staggering, angering question during and after the course. It still makes me mad. Anatomy as it is classically taught is not education at all but a socialization process. At least, it is a traditional rite of passage which physicians have experienced from the days when medical students had little to study but the organs of the body and the techniques of blood-letting. In the modern context, however, anatomy assumes a greater and more sinister significance. It is trial by memory and exposure. It is medical school's boot camp where the average youth is toughened, taught discipline, and passed along to more relevant studies with a sense of now being part of the medical fraternity. I cannot possibly remember the six, or however many, structures that pass through the carpal tunnel of the wrist, though I spent a week of my life studying them, but I do remember Granny and I do remember the professor and I have not forgotten the lessons they taught me.

Many physicians argue the merits of the anatomy experience. The demystification of death, a toughening, if you will, as well as an ability to digest and remember a huge number of facts are essential attributes of a doctor. To a degree I concur. But anatomy was destructive over-kill. It is damaging to start teaching death before the student has experienced life. It is stunting and makes one callous. Why not start medical school in the newborn nursery or on the maternity ward? Why not start in out-patient clinics or in homes or in schools? Why begin in the morgue? Similarly it is wrong to rank students, and in some cases eliminate them, on the basis of their memory. I had two classmates who fell by the wayside in the first year and anatomy was the chief stumbling block. I came very close to quitting myself—and anatomy was the primary cause.

A rigid student pecking order quickly developed, promoted largely by the Anatomy Department. Grades were posted in the lab after each exam for all to read. Good students—that is, students with good grades—were adulated. Students with mediocre or poor grades mulled their unhappy lot and hoped that by some stroke of fate they would be at the top of the list in the future. To this day I can probably name the ten best anatomy students in my class as I am sure most of my other classmates could, because the topic received so much attention in the first year of school. No one, though, could list the really good interviewers or medical historians of the class. No one could tell you who was particularly skilled at dealing with a dying patient or the family of a patient already deceased. No one knew who was compassionate or insightful, or even who was good with a scalpel and who could suture. These facts were rarely recorded and certainly never posted. Until we graduated, and even now, anyone could tell you who the good anatomy students were, but no one had any idea who was destined to be a good physician. In the absence of yardsticks, we continued to assume that the fortunate who had good memories as proven on their cadavers were the best doctors in our class.

The competitiveness, callousness, and the mindless discipline that the first year of medical school taught and that anatomy epitomized were destructive to me personally and to medical students in general. It is this brutal removal from the common paths of life that begins the mystification of the physician in his own mind and in the mind of society. Certainly, the thinking goes, anyone who has spent a year immersed in a dead human body no longer stands beside his fellows as a common laborer. He must be somehow elevated, changed by the experience. The priesthood and the military use similar techniques in training their novitiates. These techniques are entirely inappropriate to the education of any medical workers. I went to medical school to learn a skill that I could use to serve people, that would bring me closer to them. I did not decide to become a physician—and, in fairness, I think few of my classmates opted for medicine—with any expectation of elevation, beautification, or removal from my nonmedical peers.

Yet these processes were worked on us. On balance I found the first year of medicine upsetting and disappointing. During its course I frequently could not remember why I had decided to study medicine. The work was so mindless and competitive that I could see no idealism, no humanity, and no pleasure anywhere. I considered quitting half a dozen times, once going so far as to obtain a job as a teacher and hunting for an apartment to go with it. At the last minute I decided to pass up the job and stay in school for the remainder of the year. But I was not at all convinced at that point that I wanted to be a physician or that I would ever become one.

Actually, my reason for becoming a civil rights worker, for guarding the church, were not so different from those of Cat or Mr. Sills. We were all desperate in our own ways. They sought redress from economic and racial oppression; I hoped to escape the intellectual and spiritual oppression which had become my life as a would-be doctor. I needed to find some reason, some cause, to help the study of medicine make sense. Without that I would not be able to go on. It was not so much altruism that got me to the back-country church as a searching necessity that represented change in my life, just as self-defense stood out as a new step for Cat and Mr. Sills. All three of us were locked in a struggle, more with our previous lives than with the arsonists from town. The church was our stand.

During the spring of the first year of medical school I learned of the Medical Committee for Human Rights (MCHR). Founded during the summer of 1964 to provide medical support for Freedom Summer and the Civil Rights Movement, the Chicago chapter of MCHR was looking for medical students to go South for three months during the summer of 1965. They offered transportation and support ($20 per week) for volunteers who would go to Mississippi and, working with the Freedom Democratic party, begin to raise health as an issue: Why did black babies die at twice the rate of white ones? Why did whites in Mississippi live on the average ten years longer than blacks? Why were hospitals segregated? At the same time the university pushed lab jobs for students as research assistants "with the possibility of publishing." It was quite clear that the lab was not for me. I applied to MCHR and two weeks after my last anatomy exam I was on a bus headed south.

Arriving in Holmes County in the delta country of north central Mississippi I went to live with the Rust family on a dilapidated farm. Mrs. Rust (I felt like a redneck the few times I called her Magnolia) weighed a generous three hundred pounds and ruled what was left of her family with a gentle hand. Her husband had disappeared north with her eldest son some years before, sending home occasional illiterate postcards or a twenty-dollar bill. Two daughters were raising families somewhere in Illinois. To her great pride and credit she was helping a son and a daughter in their early twenties through college in Mississippi. I slept under a large Alcorn A & M pennant reminding me always of their achievement. Cat was Mrs. Rust's youngest. A muscular sixteen-year-old, he stayed at home by everybody's agreement to look after his mother and the "farm."

Mrs. Rust was a teacher. She taught third grade in the local "Attendance Center"—Mississippi shorthand for a black school. Twenty-five years before she had graduated from a black high school, a major achievement in those days, took some teacher training courses, and had been a teacher ever since. Her hand and her spelling were a seventh grader's but her enthusiasm and touch with children made her a better than average teacher by any standards. She apologized profusely and, I thought, a little bitterly for her writing and her spelling whenever she left me a note. Sweat poured from her black brow at all hours of the day or night and, though I never saw her eat much, she constantly drank from a large jar of water which she carried with her everywhere. Mrs. Rust's three-year-old grandson also lived with us. Vivacious, satin-skinned, and mischievous, he adopted me as his father and playmate. We spent many happy hours roughhousing, feeding match boxes and soap wrappers to the hogs (who loved them) and reading his one Golden Book over and over again.

A battered black vintage Chevrolet pickup served as transportation for all of us. The truck burned a quart of oil for every two gallons of gas, making it painfully expensive to drive—a tax for never having the capital to get the rings repaired. We lived in perpetual squalor. Mrs. Rust's salary came only during school months and she had no income during the summer. Cat was unemployed and I received a money order from MCHR every two weeks, half of which ($20) I immediately turned over to Mrs. Rust. For two days after that we ate well—meat, soda pop, coffee. Then we limped along for ten days on greens with ham bone and Kool-Aid, and eventually greens with no ham bone and water. The farm itself produced very little, but then very little went into it. We killed and ate an occasional chicken. The three hogs were to be butchered in the fall so we simply watched them turn garbage into flesh, an amazing phenomenon for a city boy. Cat had ambitiously planted a field of corn in the spring but had left it untended. Hopeless rows of seedy corn competed with the hardy weeds in the dry summer sun. The field failed to produce a single ear of edible corn.

The Rust family had done what many people in many communities would never have done. They bravely, gamely shared what little they had with me in the knowledge of likely reprisals. Mrs. Rust was never sure, for instance, that the school would reemploy her in the fall despite her twenty-five-year record. The thought of fire bombings, shootings, and beatings troubled the family before, during, and after my stay. Cat surely enjoyed the notoriety of driving around town with me in his pickup but he knew, and I knew, that the whites in town were calling him a no-good-civil-rights-nigger, in the past often the prelude to a lynching. Yet the family took those risks. They did it, as far as I could tell, out of a belief in their own community and a faith in change. Somebody had to house the civil rights worker and they accepted the challenge.

In the black community I became known as "the baby doctor." This had nothing to do with pediatrics but was the local interpretation of what it was to be a medical student. I was not yet a full-grown doctor but was destined to be soon. Fortunately people did not besiege me with all their medical complaints. I think there was a sense that I was not really open for business (which I was most certainly not). Yet local people took satisfaction from the presence of a medical person in their midst. It gave the community a status it had never had before. I wasn't at any gathering for long before I was pointed out as the *doctor* civil rights worker. The people had never had a doctor of their own of any sort and they were proud to have me on their side—even if I was only a "baby doctor."

By and large, I stayed away from the white community. There had never been a civil rights worker or any Movement activities in the area before and no one was sure how people would behave. We were particularly concerned about how certain hotheads ("pecker-woods," the blacks called them) would react. In filling stations, at the diner, in the pool halls there lived a demimonde of bitter, angry white men who talked obsessively of killing "niggers and nigger-lovin' whites." Luckily their only act during my stay in Holmes County was the abortive attempt to burn down the church. Generally I had little opportunity and little reason to talk to white people in town. Cat (and varying numbers of other black youths) went almost everywhere with me. One day, though, I was alone walking through the white section of town. On a residential street I passed two white girls who looked to be thirteen or fourteen. They had noticed me coming and as I walked by them they called, "Hey you! You fucker! You nigger lover!" As I turned they gave me the finger and repeated, "You fucker, you nigger lover" until I was out of earshot. Their message was clear and ugly. I was not anonymous.

At the suggestion of the local Movement people, I attempted to visit the three doctors in town and the segregated forty-bed hospital. The doctors were white and all maintained separate waiting and examination rooms for white and black patients. Two refused to see me at all, one stating flatly that since he was director of the hospital he did not want me "to put my pinko-carpetbag-ass one foot inside the hospital" or he would "do the surgery himself." I never went. The third, a Dr. Singer, agreed to see me. I wore a tie and a clean, pressed pair of corduroys when I went to visit him. Mrs. Rust later told me she had never been so proud in all her civil rights work as when "our doctor" went to visit "the white doctor" dressed like one of them. Dr. Singer was pleasant enough. He sat with me in his drab office with its twin waiting and examining rooms and assured me that he was sorry I had come to town under "these" conditions. It was a nice town, he claimed, with good people. Things were changing. They would be better in the future for both races, but for the moment people had to live the way they were accustomed. I neither challenged him nor agreed with him, feeling that my job was only to serve notice that people with some medical knowledge were monitoring the medical care given to blacks. I think he understood that but considered me, realistically enough, a minimal threat. I did ask Dr. Singer how he justified segregated facilities from a medical point of view. Did he really feel, I inquired, that different examination tables were necessary for his white and black patients? "Young man," he retorted, "you haven't been in medicine very long, nowhere as long as me. In time you'll learn a few things. One of them will be that medicine isn't science. It's people. If people don't want to be put in the same hospital room or sit in the same waiting room or get examined on the same table as nigras, I just have to go along with it. I don't make the rules people live by. I just do my job. People make the rules." "People" and "nigras" weren't the same thing to Dr. Singer and that answered my question far better than his homilies about medicine.

Toward the end of our twenty-minute visit he admonished me to be careful around town because of the "few troublemakers." "Most people in town are good people. They're exactly like people anywhere else in America, decent and lawful. But just like anywhere else, there are a few who can make trouble. You should watch out for them. But most all folks are good, law-abiding folks." As I left him I thought again, as I did frequently, of the murdered civil rights workers of the summer before and the thousand lynchings and beatings that no one ever recorded. I wondered if he was correct in saying that Mississippi was no different from any other part of America. Would communities in New Hampshire or Iowa or Oregon condone or conceal vigilantes in their midst? Many of the problems I observed for the first time in 1965 (racism, dead-end schooling, wage slavery, and so forth) I took to be unique to the South. I have since observed variations of the same conditions in many parts of the United States, and I would certainly not argue now, as I might have then, that the North is right and the South is wrong. Yet I still think Dr. Singer was wrong. There is something special about the tight, time-honored racism of the whites in a small southern town. It is not the violence itself that is unique. Racist beatings, bombings, and murder have occurred in the North. But I cannot imagine a town of a thousand or five thousand where many people know the facts of violence without somebody coming forward to protest. In most communities in America there is sufficient diversity so that a reservoir of dissent always exists. In the South it did not. The social glue of racism was too strong. No one ever came forward from the white community to express anger at the attempt to burn a church. Dr. Singer had not the slightest inclination to take a stand against segregation in his office or his hospital.

Although the visit to Dr. Singer proved to be my only formal contact with the local medical community, much of my time in Mississippi was spent working on health problems. Unfortunately nothing in my first year of medical school had prepared me for work as a rural health officer. I had been taught the structures of the carpal tunnel (perhaps I still remembered them then) and the chemicals secreted by the neurohypophysis, but no first aid, no public health techniques, and no methods of health education. The model for American medical school training was (and is) predominantly private practice. Public health, first aid, and the like do not generally concern the private practitioner and isoenzymes, vectorcardiography, and organ transplants are much more the style. Public health is for "emerging" nations and the history books. So I began my work as a medical organizer with common sense and a few days of orientation by MCHR as my only assets. My initial goal was to set up a Health Association in the nearby town to get people talking about their medical problems. With the help of the Freedom Democratic party I convened the first meeting at the home of Mrs. Viola Summers, a very proper, elderly black woman. Mrs. Summers, a veteran of church activities, opened and closed the meeting with a prayer. In place of a hymn, however, we sang a spirited "We Shall Overcome." The fact that this was the first civil rights meeting actually held in the town made everybody tense. Mr. Winters stood at the door watching the street during the entire session. When we were finished, there was an air of jubilation in the group because we had really succeeded in having a civil rights meeting, a free meeting in town. That sense was certainly more important than any medical information that changed hands.

At first people declined to talk, stating that they had come to see what troubled everybody else. At length a woman in the group spoke angrily of her recent experience as a patient at the local hospital. That was sufficient. Much of the rest of the evening was consumed by people heatedly trading tales about the hospital and the local physicians. A number of stories were confused, disjointed, or were clear misunderstandings. But their significance was that they were told at all and that the group listened and responded supportively. To a person, they resented the segregated facilities they faced everywhere they went. They were particularly angry at one doctor who systematically refused to see patients who had any outstanding bills. This practice, more than any other, hurt the black community. Generally poor, constrained by a seasonal agricultural income, many blacks had difficulty making payments on time. It was one thing to default a payment on a television set, the Health Association thought, and lose it, but it was quite another to be refused medical care. To them, the denial of services by a man living well (one of the largest houses in town and a Cadillac) to a man in pain because of an outstanding debt of $5 was an outrage. Their anger was compounded because they recognized an important fact about medicine in a small town—it was a closed market. The doctor with the Cadillac had not only the skill to help them but he had absolute say-so as to whom he would help. There were no competing brands. If he refused to see a patient for bad debts, the other two doctors would generally follow suit. There was no court of appeal and no immediate alternative.

After several meetings the Health Association decided on a course of action. They had learned through an NAACP lawyer that the new civil rights law made it illegal to maintain segregated facilities in hospitals constructed with the assistance of federal money. The local hospital had been built and expanded with the help of federal Hill–Burton funds. Therefore, under Mrs. Summers's leadership the group decided to send a delegation to the hospital administrator to ask that the segregated wings of the hospital be merged and that the differential in wages for black and white employees be eliminated. At the last meeting of the Health Association that I attended the delegation reported its experiences. They had met with the hospital administrator accompanied by the doctor who wanted to do surgery on me and the town sheriff wearing his hat and gun. The three white men had looked upset, which gave heart to the delegation. The administrator responded to their charges by explaining that the hospital had been arranged the way it was so that everybody would be happiest. "Some nigra folks," he told the austere Mrs. Summers, "don't like being mixed with white folks. This civil rights talk has your head all confused." Mrs. Summers answered that the "civil rights talk" was there to stay and that next time they would come back with their lawyer. When they left the administrator was furious.

Despite the meager results, the Health Association was delighted with the attack. Each member of the delegation told his version of the story to the mirth of all present. At length, the association decided to get in touch with the NAACP lawyer and file formal notice with the hospital that it was in violation of the law. Two years later, after many legal battles, the hospital facility was desegregated.

As a spinoff of the Health Association I was invited to a neighboring town to give a class in sex education for a group of teenagers. My contact was a young woman from that community who had been away at college for one year and learned about birth control. She was worried about her young sisters and felt the information would generally benefit the community. I arrived, equipped with a condom purchased at a local drug store and a half-used pack of birth-control pills borrowed from a civil rights worker, to find a giggling group of girls ranging from my twenty-year-old hostess down to her eleven-year-old sister. There wasn't a male present beside myself. We gathered in a large group on the porch of a house. My recollection is that there were girls everywhere—on the steps, on the railings, in front of me and behind me. Most were laughing. When we started, though, they became serious, listening to me talk about the anatomy of the sexual organs. That much I knew from Granny. They asked some good questions and paid careful attention to everything I said. I had begun to discuss birth control, passing my gadgets around the group, when the giggling began again. Surely it was my fault, I thought. I tried to remain poised and continue talking as I searched for the cause of the new laughter. I noticed one of the girls point and I glanced behind me to discover that the man of the house, the father of my hostess and her sisters, had pulled his chair up behind the screen door and was sitting listening to the session. Dozens of contradictory thoughts passed through my head. Was he angry or pleased? Did he think birth control was a good idea or not? Did he know what birth control was? Did he think this white man had come here to teach his children promiscuity or, to the contrary, was this white man teaching black genocide, peddling his contraceptive devices? It didn't matter much because my decision about carrying on the class was being made for me—it was dissolving in front of me. The pills and the condom had been hurriedly returned and the young women were slipping away. I never did find out what the father thought for he too had disappeared from behind the door. I taught no more sex education classes after that and my half-completed birth-control lecture still remains to be finished. It matters little now because the youngest of the girls there is already in her twenties and, I am afraid, the die is cast.

Later that night a half moon came out making the road and the clearing in front of the church visible. Cat woke up and I smoked some of his cigarettes to help time pass. Occasionally we could hear trucks gearing up on the Jackson to Memphis highway some three miles distant through the woods or the sound of the freight engines switching boxcars on the Illinois Central tracks in town. Sitting guard, we eavesdropped on American commerce. I wondered what the truckers or the trainmen would think of us protecting a church with shotguns. Would they be on our side or would they think we deserved whatever we got in the way of trouble? Would they do the same in their communities for some cause of theirs? Would they care at all? It seemed absurd to be so close to the mainstream of America—industry, technology, transportation—doing something as medieval as guarding a church with a gun. Yet we were not in the mainstream. I had to keep telling myself that. Perhaps I was raised in the mainstream and I was training to be a doctor in the mainstream, but the Movement was outside of the mainstream. In Mississippi I was no longer at the head of the class, scion of the powerful, son of the New Frontier. To whites, to doctors, to the establishment, I was despicable. I was part of the black community and, worse, I was a troublemaker, an agitator, a nigger lover, a commie. From the vantage point of the Mississippi woods those trucks and trains sounded different. The American mainstream looked less reasonable, less equitable, and less safe.

America had not done well by Mr. Sills and Cat Rust nor had it been generous to Magnolia Rust or Viola Summers or the dozens of other black Mississippians I lived and worked with during the summer of 1965. They were poorly schooled, ill fed and badly cared for in a generally wealthy country. Knowing this, a simple choice presented itself in my mind: either their poverty resulted from their being black and, therefore, inadequate (the racist explanation), or their poverty derived from their being black and therefore segregated, exploited, and oppressed. While I was in Mississippi I saw enough to persuade me forever that the squalor of the black community was caused by the system and not the people. The Mississippi system foreordained the poverty of blacks. To overcome that poverty the system had to be changed and that was a struggle which had become very important for me. In Holmes County, in the Civil Rights Movement, I experienced a cause and felt a love that helped medicine make sense to me. The Movement needed what I had to offer. It was no longer irrelevant how well I did in school; I had people to work for, people who needed what I could learn. In the woods of Mississippi, away from the medical center, far away from the labs and lecture halls, well outside the standard avenues of medical approbation, I discovered why I wanted to be a doctor.

When the sun came up, Mr. Sills said good-by and walked up the road. Cat and I walked in the other direction down the road toward his farm. A rooster crowed, dogs barked, and I felt very tired.

2

Student of the Body, Captive of the System

The first two years of medical school passed very slowly, years when it was rumored there were real people with real diseases and not just test tubes, experimental dogs, and cadavers. One friend insisted after every new disease he studied that they wouldn't be making it anymore by the time he was ready to treat it. Occasionally I would find some excuse to walk the hospital corridors away from our labs and scrutinize the men and women in white darting in and out of rooms everywhere.

In the spring quarter of the second year, we were sent onto the hospital floors for the first time to see patients, as part of a Physical Diagnosis course. Indeed, it was the first time we examined living people with our own hands, the first time we were called "Doctor," and, perhaps most important, the first time we wore our white coats. The last was most significant because it was most tangible. We felt awkward examining patients and I always looked around to see whom they were talking to when the nurses called me "Doctor." But there was no denying the white coat. It looked authentic and it felt authentic. It took apparent teenagers and turned them into physicians. It took acne-ridden fraternity boys and transformed them into surgeons, internists, and pediatricians. I remember being well pleased with its above-the-knee length and its deep pockets that easily accommodated a stethoscope, leaving the ear pieces to bob importantly above the pocket lip.

The students, it turned out, weren't the only people interested in style. The medical school administration was highly concerned with their students' grooming and attire. The year was 1966 and beards were still considered by many to be the domain of those they chose to call hippies. Facial hair was clearly a coming commodity among young people and two classmates sported nicely trimmed beards through the first year and a half of medical school. We speculated a good deal about what would happen if they didn't shave before they started Physical Diagnosis. At that time no third- or fourth-year medical students and not a single member of the clinical faculty wore a beard. The stage was set for a challenge. One of my hirsute colleagues avoided the problem by shaving, while the other held his ground. Sure enough, in the second week of the quarter he received a terse note from the Dean of Students requesting him to shave. The news of the demand spread quickly through the class, angering many people. To me the note stood as an affront, a threat to my individuality. I wasn't wearing a beard at the time nor did I have any particular intention of wearing one, but the idea that some medical school bureaucrat could dictate my hair style and dress as well as what I studied and how many hours of my life I spent in the hospital and how I spent my summers infuriated me. I was already tortured by the wrenching change in discipline and life style that medicine demanded. Somehow the command that Jim Waller shave his beard was the last straw, the unacceptable excess in the invasion of my privacy as a human being.

Looking back on it now, the SWAB (Save WAller's Beard) campaign seems amusing but hardly political. At the time, though, the episode had a compelling importance for me and, I think, for a number of the others who participated in it. Inconsequential as it might seem, the fight was for the individual and the rights of the individual against the encroachments of the institution—the institution of medicine as embodied in the medical school. Patients, the dean claimed, could not relate comfortably to doctors with beards; therefore, beards had to go. Was it our job, we countered, was it our responsibility to set every patient at ease no matter what the personal price? Did he mean we had to be paunchy, forty-five, and balding to practice reasonable medicine? More significantly, did we have to be male and white (as almost all of us were) to become acceptable physicians? No, no, the dean spluttered. You are blowing the issue completely out of context. Being clean-shaven is simply a courtesy to the patients who entrust themselves to our care. We cannot offend them.

I didn't buy his argument, nor did the majority of my classmates. After a week or two of debate, during which time Waller stalwartly refused to take a razor to his now-famous face, some two-thirds of the class signed the SWAB petition *requesting* the permission of the medical school for Waller to remain as he was—neat and bearded. Eventually the issue was referred to the chief of the first clinical service on which Waller was scheduled to work, Internal Medicine. The head of the department was a curt Swiss-German. The question was raised in a departmental meeting and reportedly caused an angry debate. Students, of course, were not present. Allegedly the European professor listened to the heated deliberations without saying anything and, at length, ended the discussion saying, "Beards, schmeards, if the boy knows his medicine he'll pass. That's all there is to it."

So Waller kept his beard, which he wears proudly to this day. The class was elated by the victory and I personally felt that we had struck a blow for human, or at least medical, liberty.

Today, in honesty, I am not so sure. The SWAB campaign was, at that time, profoundly political for me. Waller's beard was a symbol of departure from medical style that was oppressive and exclusionary. The fight to save it represented not just a battle for individualism, but an effort to liberalize a tight and arbitrary medical norm. For me, beards became an insignia. They indicated resistance to blind tradition and thoughtless authority. Beards were in themselves political and the sign of a political person. Now, the better part of a decade later, beards, long hair, dashikis, sandals, and the like can be found in medical schools as they can be found elsewhere on campus. They have long since ceased to be the domain of people interested in change. They are a style in themselves, often worn by the most self-satisfied and complacent. Now I am a little embarrassed by the fervor and religiosity with which we carried out the SWAB campaign. But it remains an important point of departure for my own political thinking as well as that of Waller and a number of our classmates.

Fresh from the SWAB victory, I ventured onto my first clinical rotation. There I encountered a dozen new occupations that were destined to become part of my daily life as a physician—rounds, grand rounds, and roundsmanship; charting and chart review; interns and residents and attendings* and the pros and cons of each; blood drawing, urinalysis, rectal exams, and so on.

---

* The terms referring to the various categories of physicians in teaching hospitals can be confusing. An "attending physician" or an "attending" is a senior doctor of faculty rank who is in charge of a medical unit (a ward or a service). Most often he or she is a recognized, board-certified specialist in the appropriate specialty area—pediatrics, internal medicine, surgery, and so forth. A "resident physician" or a "resident" is a graduate M.D. with several years of training experience. A "chief resident" is the most senior resident on a given service who often has special teaching or leadership responsibilities. An "intern" is a physician in training in his or her first year out of medical school.

Above all and at last there were patients. My first one—whom I will always remember vividly—was a garrulous fifty-five-year-old musician. (Let me apologize for the use of the word "my" to refer to the patient. "My patient," "my case," and "my diagnosis" are possessive, egocentric traditions of medical speech to which I have grown accustomed. In no way do I intend to infringe upon the individuality and the rights of any people with whom I have worked. Most patients, and this one in particular, remain very much their own people in spite of verbal and physical assaults by the medical profession.) The musician entered the University of Chicago Hospital with a staggering string of complaints including headache, blurred vision, insomnia, constipation, gas pains, and tremors. The last was his most aggravating problem since he was a concert violinist and tremors did not go well with his art.

As with most patients entering university hospitals, he immediately inherited a team of skilled, somewhat skilled, and in this case, unskilled doctors to watch over him during his stay. Our team consisted of a well-versed attending physician in charge of the entire hospital floor, a resident with three or four years of medical experience under his belt, an intern, and myself, as yet two long years from graduation, gamely approaching my first living patient. My job as the student was to perform the first and most exhaustive medical history and physical exam on the violinist, Mr. Gamoretz.

The complete medical history that is supposed to be memorized and administered by medical students varies little from hospital to hospital. It is a meticulous and sobering affair designed to seek out information about nosebleeds, number of trips to the bathroom in the average night, occupation, amount of coffee consumed, maternal and grandmaternal breast cancer, sexual problems, and the color and consistency of any sputum coughed up, among other things. In the Physical Diagnosis course we had rehearsed taking medical histories on each other and on an occasional, already well-examined, patient. Mr. Gamoretz was my first attempt from scratch. For the occasion I had miniaturized the eight-page medical history questionnaire that we had been given, transcribing it in tiny print onto a single sheet. I planned to use the sheet to unobtrusively check the answers to some two hundred questions I would casually ask Mr. Gamoretz.

With the sheet lashed to a clipboard and held in a sweaty hand, carrying a small black bag of newly acquired medical instruments, wearing a freshly starched white coat, I walked down the long corridor to the violinist's room. "Hello, Mr. Gamoretz. I am Doctor Mullan. I will be one of your doctors while you are here. If you don't mind I would like to ask you a few questions about what's troubling you."

"Well first of all young man, get yourself a chair and sit down. There are some things I want to tell you." The "young man" part almost killed me but I got the chair. "If I weren't Jewish I'd be a Christian Scientist. As a matter of fact, I'm sort of a Jewish Scientist. Do you know what that means? That means I don't believe in doctors or in medicines. I suppose I'll have to listen to what you have to say, but don't expect me to believe any of it. I'm here because my wife told me she'd throw me out of the house if I didn't come, not because I want to be. My head hurts, my stomach won't act right, and my hands shake when they shouldn't. But that's not why I'm here. I'm here because Alice says so. Is that clear?"

The palm print on the single sheet on my clipboard was positively wet now. "Well, that's pretty clear, Mr. Gamoretz. I would like to ask you a little more about your headaches, if I could."

"And another thing. I'm a vegetarian. I have been for the last thirty years. It's the reason I'm in such good health. The lunch tray they brought me had meat and the vegetables were terrible. Overcooked, stringy, canned, and awful. What can I do to get my regular, healthy diet?"

Even now I find it staggering; my first patient was a vegetarian, "Jewish Scientist" violinist, in the hospital, according to him, because his wife sent him. In fact, he was a great deal more affable, more worried, and sicker than our first interchange suggested. In many ways he was a good first patient. It turned out that he liked to talk about himself, which helped in the administration of my voluminous, not-so-casual medical history. We spent much of the afternoon discussing the ins and outs of his health in great detail. At length I examined him, a fifteen-minute anticlimax after the hours of history taking.

Sitting at the Formica desk at the Nursing Station after leaving Mr. Gamoretz, I felt very discouraged. I had done what they said. I administered a laborious history and a careful physical exam. I now knew the man's eating, drinking, smoking, and sexual habits. I had looked in his eyes, listened to his heart, palpated his liver and put a finger in his rectum. Somehow I expected that, all this done, I would have reached a new plane of understanding. It seemed only reasonable that some mysterious diagnosis or series of diagnoses would have been revealed to me. Instead, I fingered the notes on my clipboard and reflected on my insight into Mr. Gamoretz—a talkative middle-aged musician, with high blood pressure. That, it appeared, was all I had learned from a three-hour exercise of my new skills and my new instruments and that was no more than any nurse or orderly or, in fact, anyone off the street taught to take a blood pressure could have deduced in far less time. What had two years in medical school, two tough disciplined years done for me? Had I been such a poor student that I had learned nothing? Or was this all there was to medicine, some common sense and some long names, such as hypertension instead of high blood pressure?

One of the enduring strong points of medical education in this country is that it is built on the apprenticeship system. The student in most medical school services spends the largest percentage of time with and undoubtedly learns the most from the intern. The intern, in turn, learns from the resident, the resident from the chief resident, and the chief resident from the attending. This system is extremely hierarchical and invites the abuses of all hierarchies, but the basic locked-step, personal, experiential method of teaching has been, in my experience, both effective and gratifying. The intern, after all, has the best sense of what the student is going through since he is separated from his own studenthood by only a few months. The resident knows the trials of becoming an intern because he has been through it only recently. And so forth.

Late that first afternoon my own apprenticeship as a clinical medical student began. I was fortunate in sharing Mr. Gamoretz with an astute and sensitive intern named Swartz. He also had met and examined Mr. Gamoretz and he found me wallowing in self-pity and contempt. He took the time to sit down with me and review my findings and my discouragement. In fact I had missed some subtle points in the exam—the changes in the small vessels in the back of the eye and the extra sound in the heart that developed the case for hypertension and suggested the severity of the disease process. But, on balance, his conclusions were the same as mine: Mr. Gamoretz was a difficult, likeable man with severe hypertension that could account for a number of his other complaints. He praised my workup, pointing out how much information I had gotten that could be of potential benefit in treating Mr. Gamoretz. More important, he encouraged me to be satisfied with what I had diagnosed. "Every patient isn't hiding a case of Rocky Mountain spotted fever or Tse-Tse syndrome," he argued. "Common illnesses *are* common. We should be happy for that because most of us wouldn't make the esoteric diagnoses anyway. Just because somebody else can make the diagnosis of elevated blood pressure, your work isn't invalidated. Diagnosis isn't the whole job anyway. You have a lot more work to do. You have to find out what's causing it and you have to treat it." He was right about that because I had little idea where to turn next to further test and treat Mr. Gamoretz's illness.

I felt a great deal better after our talk. In the subsequent days, under Swartz's tutelage, I learned much about how to work up and treat hypertension. My initial quandary, however, taught me a lesson that has stayed with me, although I appreciated it very little at the time. There is no quantum difference between the skills or insights of a physician and those of any other skilled observer, whatever the credentials. Although I had never lived in any particular awe of medicine, I did expect that when I began my practice as a doctor I would suddenly experience and see things in a significantly different way. Naïvely, perhaps, I anticipated a sudden burst of wisdom, a sudden view from behind the stethoscope that would drastically change my powers of observation and evaluation. Quite reasonably no such change occurred.

And yet many people believe this change takes place and, certainly, many doctors behave as though it has. I firmly believe a person's skills in medicine, as elsewhere, are based on natural ability, rigor of training, and length of experience. Obviously there were many nurses in the hospital who would have been more skilled in diagnosing and, I daresay, in treating Mr. Gamoretz than I was. That thought was unacceptable to me at that time because I felt that a doctor—even a student doctor—should be sharper than any other medical worker. It was indeed threatening to me that a nurse could diagnose an illness as well as or better than I could. That notion, that medical chauvinism, is deeply rooted in our society as it was in me and is a recurrent obstacle in the way of developing new patterns of health care in this country.

In the days that followed, Mr. Gamoretz was explored in every way. His body was invaded by proctoscopes, needles, and X-rays. No effort was spared in collecting and studying his bodily fluids. His kidneys were visualized, his stool impounded, and his already grim vegetarian diet mutilated. In the end his diagnosis was quite similar to what we had started with: "essential hypertension"—significant blood-pressure elevation without other contributing cause.

Fortunately there are a number of effective medications for the reduction of blood pressure, but treating the affable violinist proved no easy feat. It developed that Mr. Gamoretz had been treated for hypertension several years earlier. His previous physician had tried a number of different antihypertensive agents, none of which had worked. The musician had, by his own report, chewed all the pills he had been offered and rejected those whose taste he didn't like. He argued that his years of experience with health foods enabled him to determine which pills would be effective and which would not and most antihypertensives were "gut rot." As we began our attempt at treatment once again, he taste-tested all the medication offered. Only reserpine, a time-honored but weak antihypertensive, was to his liking. After a week or so of coaxing, pleading, and threatening by various members of the white-coat team, Mr. Gamoretz went home. He carried with him three prescriptions, one of which (reserpine) he promised to use while he agreed to consider the other two. His hands shook less and, despite our physical and verbal assaults on him, his blood pressure was somewhat decreased. As he and his wife left the floor, they stopped to say good-by to me. He was friendly and chatty as always and invited me to come to his house when I had a free evening. "I'll fix you a roast, a vegetable roast, the likes of which you've never tasted. Once you've had it you'll never go back to meat. A roast with gravy."

As with virtually all the patients whose lives I briefly shared as a medical student, I heard no more from Mr. Gamoretz. He probably returned to one clinic or another at the medical center (he was certainly invited back) but medical education emphasizes disease and not relationship and no provisions are made to follow patients you have come to know. He was, indeed, a good first patient. His idiosyncrasies were, perhaps, a bit far-fetched, but he was a paradigm of the man-meets-medical-system problem. It is simple to work out a schedule for pill taking, dieting, alcohol abstention and the like but it is never easy to integrate such regimens into the lives of people. The gap between medical planning—even reasonable medical planning—and what is called "patient compliance" is huge. Mr. Gamoretz was a study in vocal noncompliance. Between the scientific precision of the examinations performed on him and the final, futile efforts to lower his blood pressure stood a vast chasm populated by attitudes, beliefs, and habits—humanness. The most advanced science in a university medical center was not sufficient to help Mr. Gamoretz nor is it sufficient, by itself, to benefit most people. That, more than the diagnosis and treatment of hypertension, is what I carried away from my experience with the vegetarian violinist.

But I soon learned clinical medicine wasn't all dealing with people. There was a constant demand for manual skills which had to be learned awkwardly, one by one. No textbook written could adequately explain how to start an I.V., draw blood, or do a spinal tap. These tasks had to be taught patiently by the intern to the faltering student. The real hero of the situation was often the unsuspecting patient who had to endure the second or third needle stick or the uncomfortably prolonged procedure.

My most awkward moment came not with a patient at all but with a mouse. For decades the diagnosis of pneumococcal pneumonia (a common form of pneumonia) was made by injecting a thimble full of sputum coughed up by the sick individual into the belly of a healthy, innocent mouse. It is a practice now largely and properly abandoned but in the early days of bacteriology it was one of the surest techniques for diagnosing the serious ailment. Mice, it turns out, are exquisitely sensitive to the pneumococcus and after twelve hours or so an investigation of the lining of the belly of the dead or dying mouse will reveal indisputable signs if the germ if present. For reasons of tradition, as far as I can tell, the University of Chicago was still teaching and using this technique in the mid-1960s.

The exercise required some knowledge of rodent technology—a knowledge I did not possess and the sort of thing one cannot handily look up in any textbooks lying around the hospital. So late one evening my friend Swartz handed me a specimen bottle three fingers deep with two-tone (green and white) lumpy liquid and told me to take it over to the lab and run a mouse test, I was at a loss. I knew the theory of the test but I had no idea how to convey the semi-solid fluid into the poor animal's innards. The lab was a small cubicle stocked with a variety of microbiological tools (a Bunsen burner, syringes, specimen plates, and so on) and two walls lined with cages full of mice. Both the cubicle and the larger lab next door were vacant and there was no one to consult as to what to do next. I hadn't asked Swartz for any hints because his matter-of-fact attitude in handing me the bottle suggested that the test was a simple one that anybody could do. After all I had completed two years of medical science. Surely the mouse test must have been covered there; but I could not remember anything about dealing with mice.

Cautiously, gamely, I drew a milliliter or two of the greenish sputum into a syringe and attached a small needle. I studied the cages, searching for a mouse that looked reasonable, that appeared sympathetic and might be able to understand my quandary. They all looked about the same. At length I picked a little fellow in a big cage. I placed him on the counter, cage and all, and reviewed the situation. Clearly I had to remove him from his cage, turn him on his back and stab his tummy with my needle to deliver the payload. The prime question, though, was how to grab him and hold him to accomplish the chore. I didn't know then as I know now (Swartz showed me later) that holding a mouse by the tail and pulling him causes him to resist and stretch out so that he can be collared firmly by the back and neck and then abused in whatever manner necessary. Instead I bravely grabbed him as he cowered in one corner of his cage. It took only the length of time for my swiftly moving, scared hand to pass out of the cage over the counter before he sank his small, sharp, white teeth into the flesh of my thumb. I yelped and slammed him on the counter, half in fear and half in anger.

The deed did not agree with him. He lay there stunned, a grey ball of fur twitching occasionally. Opportunist that I was, I ignored the pain in my thumb to take advantage of my sudden windfall—the mouse was out cold and injecting him was no longer a problem. Quickly I rammed the foul material into his belly and dropped him back in the cage. I cleaned the tiny wound on my hand, labeled his cage appropriately and waited to see if he would wake up. He did in a minute or two and I left him to find Swartz and report my victory and my breakthrough in animal technology. I felt fairly smug.

Swartz was not amused by my achievements. "Suppose the mouse has rabies. There are rabid mice, you know. If that sputum has pneumococcus in it he'll be dead by morning and we'll never know. You should have just set him aside in his cage and used another mouse." The possibility of getting a series of painful rabies shots because we could not determine the state of health of the mouse who would be dead was distressing.

"Our only choice now," Swartz continued, "is to treat the mouse against the pneumococcus and try to save him." The notion was ludicrous but sensible. We had to return to the animal lab with a syringe full of penicillin and attempt life-saving antibiosis on an eight-ounce mouse to discover if he had rabies or not. This time Swartz went with me. Wise as he was about how to handle mice and transport them in and out of their cages he, like so many of us, had never treated a mouse before. We had no idea what a mouse dose of penicillin was but attempted a reasonable guess by calculating one three-hundredth of an adult dose. The quantity of penicillin proved to be very small and hard to measure and the syringe was not properly calibrated for so small an amount. In retrospect it is altogether possible that the mouse got five to ten times as much medication as intended.

Under Swartz's skilled guidance I removed the ill-looking mouse from his cage, using the correct technique, and slowly injected the penicillin into his already punctured abdomen. We placed him back in his cage and watched him carefully. It took about fifteen seconds before it began. The mouse reared up on his rigid hind legs, turned a full circle twice and fell to the floor of the cage with giant spasms that lasted for two or three minutes before all motion ceased. "Well," concluded Swartz, "either we overdosed him or he was allergic to penicillin."

The director of the lab autopsied the mouse in the morning and assured me that there was no chance of rabies. I felt relieved and Swartz and I had a few good laughs about the situation. I am still no expert on mice (and fortunately don't have to be) but even now I remember well how to remove a mouse from a cage, how to treat the pneumococcus and what happens in penicillin overdose.

The single element of clinical medicine that surprised me the most was rounds. Rounds, for those not versed in hospitalese, are the once-daily, or twice-daily, or thrice-daily visit of the team to the patient. Of course I knew about rounds and I expected to make them from time to time. I had no idea, though, what a chunk would suddenly be taken out of my life for interminable hallway or bedside chats, for rounds generally represent the fulcrum of the teaching program in the clinical years of medical school. Every day every patient would be presented (introduced and situation updated) by the student or intern and discussed at length by the resident or attending. In retrospect it was a perfectly reasonable, important way to spend time in medical school since I probably learned more there than I did anywhere else. But it is not the image that comes to mind when one thinks of the excitement of an action-packed career in medicine; it is not the scene that one usually encounters on the nightly television medical drama. Rounds were cumbersome, meticulous, and frequently dull.

We learned soon there were certain basic concepts essential to coping with rounds. For the most part we grasped principles quickly and put them to work for ourselves, adapting like chameleons. Survival, not to say learning, depended on stamina and energy conservation. It is no easy trick to take a three-hundred-foot walk in three hours. Torpor sets in. We learned to lean against anything—walls, beds, standing trays, oxygen tanks. The optimal place to achieve support was the buttock because it came closest to sitting. Next best was the flat of the back and third, but by no means insignificant, were the hands where considerable support could be gained. Leaning forward, elbows locked, hands on a bed rail became a favorite position.

The next task was paying attention or, failing that, appearing to pay attention. Both had their place because you learned what you listened to but you were often marked on how well you participated on rounds. At least the semblance of interest and involvement were important at all times. I made a rule for myself that when my mind wandered off and I caught myself I would rivet my attention on the attending's, or the patient's Adam's apple (thyroid cartilage to us) for as long as I could, part as punishment and part as cover.

Once survival had been attended to, we concentrated our energies on what we came to call "roundsmanship." The concept of roundsmanship turned on the fact that rounds were in theory if not always in fact a hierarchical exercise. The cases were presented by the student or the intern to the senior physician present, who would determine the nature and the length of discussion of each patient. Without fail, everyone present had ulterior motives regarding the contents of rounds. The student, for instance, wanted an opportunity to show off the facts he had learned in a medical journal the night before. Another student, perhaps, would hope to avoid a long discussion of one of his patients because he knew little or nothing about the patient's disease. The intern, most likely, was anxious to see the early end of rounds because he had a new patient to admit, a dozen bloods to draw, and a hundred orders to write before he could try to catch up on the sleep he missed the night before. And so forth.

Roundsmanship was the important art of making these things happen. Roundsmanship was the clever, or occasionally not so clever, insertion of the name of last night's medical journal into the discussion of patient ailments. "Well Blevins of Harvard (very important) writing in the *New England Journal* (a good one) of two weeks ago (as if you read it every week) said that lysosmal mitochondria . . ." Roundsmanship was also the significant skill of cutting short the discussion of your patient with systemic lupus erythematosus (about which you knew little) by focusing on body rashes (a topic about which you knew a little something). You hoped the professor would amble on to your next patient when the debate about rashes ceased, leaving your ignorance of lupus undisturbed. Roundsmanship was the stealth of an intern sliding toward the next bed while still discussing the last patient in the hope that the crowd and the attending might follow.

By speaking lightly of rounds I don't mean to belittle their importance in patient care or medical education. Rounds are, as I have suggested, the bulwark of clinical teaching in a medical school setting and an essential activity in the practice of medicine. It was on rounds one day, shortly after the Gamoretz episode, that I first heard rales. Rales are the crackling noises heard in the chest of a patient suffering fluid in the lung. Its most common causes are pneumonia and heart failure. Rales are an ancient and cardinal sign in physical diagnosis. In the present epoch of autoanalyzers of the blood and space-age X-ray techniques, rales remain a simple physical sign which the human being with the aid of a stethoscope can detect and can act on. We had read about rales in our Physical Diagnosis course and were well versed in their importance but I had never actually heard them. The experience was electrifying. Suddenly the book, the abstraction, the concept came to life and surprisingly, I remember thinking, it was just as they said it would be—like tissue paper being crumpled. Elsewhere on rounds I felt a spleen for the first time—a normally sequestered organ that can be palpated only when diseased. Similarly, with the careful coaching of an attending physician, I saw papilledema—the ballooning of the back of an eye due to increased pressure in the brain. These were concrete, graphic, exciting events that I remember vividly and they all took place on rounds. While the daily stroll with the team could be tedious, it remained a key exercise in the apprenticeship of medicine.

But there were certain topics that the apprenticeship dealt with poorly, if at all. While doing my surgical clerkship, I helped care for a middle-aged man who had had part of his aorta (the largest blood vessel in the body carrying blood from the heart to the lower extremities) replaced by a synthetic tube. The lower portion of his own aorta had suffered advanced atherosclerosis—fatty clots that plugged the artery and prevented adequate blood flow to the legs. The deterioration of function in his legs forced the surgeons to remove a foot-long section of his own aorta and replace it with a plastic cylinder sewn artfully into the healthy ends of the remaining artery. All this had happened some six months previously, well before I had become a student surgeon. In the weeks before his final hospitalization signs began to develop that all was not well. One of his legs became numb and then noticeably cold. He experienced spiking fevers and pain low in his abdomen. When we hospitalized him it was clear that his artery graft was infected and at least partially clotted. Our strategy was to give him high doses of antibiotics in an effort to stem the infection prior to opening his belly a second time to shore up the graft.

At three in the morning of his second hospital day I was called (as the lowest member of the team and therefore the first up) by the floor nurse who reported that my patient's fever was up and his blood pressure falling. I took one look at him and called for help. He breathed rapidly and shallowly, sweat beaded his pale face, and his belly was board hard. We took him to the Operating Room as soon as we could assemble enough people to proceed. We ran blood into his arm as fast as it would flow. Thirty minutes after the nurse called me, three of us (the chief resident, the resident, and myself) had our hands deep in his bloody abdomen. The graft was indeed infected. As a result the adjacent wall of the natural vessel had been eroded and all at once gave way, allowing fresh blood from the heart to pump vigorously and aimlessly out among his intestines.

We could neither stem the tide of blood nor replace it fast enough to match the amount that was squirting out of his aorta, bubbling through the wound in his abdomen, running down the fronts of our green surgical gowns onto the floor. After a frantic half hour we quit. The EKG monitor reporting on the condition of the patient's heart signaled that we had lost and further efforts would be futile. The anesthesiologist turned off the blood that was still flowing and left. The resident and the chief resident followed suit, asking me to sew up the gash that ran from the chest to the pubis so the body could be taken to the morgue.

It was an eerie time. I stood over the body, the new student, fresh out of the laboratories and the textbooks of basic science, the low man on the team suddenly in charge of the high temple of the hospital—the Operating Room. I had an efficient, sterile scrub nurse waiting to hand me sutures, forceps, and scissors. The monitor was still flashing. An orderly stood obsequiously along the wall prepared to fetch anything I might command. And the patient, my patient, lay waiting, his entrails staring at me.

The body turned cold while I worked. The intestines, which I had been holding this way and that since the beginning of our labors, remained slightly warm, but the skin soon grew clammy. To me this was much stronger evidence than the EKG that the man had died.

I toiled diligently closing the rent abdomen. I was his final doctor and I felt he deserved my best. Like all students of surgery, I had practiced suturing by throwing stitches into towels, sheets, and spare cloths. Under the careful supervision of a resident I had put two stitches in a boy's forehead in the Emergency Room but I had never really put thread in anyone on my own. Now I had the entire Operating Room and two feet of a man's belly to close up. I worked as carefully and as rapidly as I could, hoping the nurse wouldn't think I was clumsy. Of course it didn't matter a great deal how accurate or how cosmetic I was since no one would ever again be looking at my patient's stomach. But I cared, and I owed him the best of what my practice with towels had taught me.

When I had finished and walked out and down the long Operating Room corridor toward the changing room, I suddenly felt faint. I sat down on a stretcher and watched the skyline brighten over the scruffy rooftops of Chicago's South Side. I had seen death before; I had attended autopsies; and goodness knows I had lived with Granny for the better part of a year. But I had never been so intimately involved with death physically as I had with the man I had just sewn up. I thought about his wife, whom I had met, and his children, who were my age. Before I went briefly to bed some six hours earlier, I had stopped in his room and chatted with him. Now the touch of his tepid guts was in my mind and his blood was matted on the front of my green surgical pajamas. I felt frightened and nauseated.

Perhaps it is impossible to teach about death. Certainly as a subject it is different from most of the scientific topics that I had labored over in school up to that point. But between anatomy and Physical Diagnosis, between cellular structure and rales, nothing much, nothing of importance had been said about death. There had been a conditioning process, to be sure, that included dissection of rats, cats, and dogs as well as the intensive exposure to the cadaver in the anatomy lab. But nowhere had we sat down to talk about the real meaning of death and dying. The precipitate and bloody death of my patient that night broke through my conditioning and left me trembling on that stretcher in the empty hallway in the Chicago dawn.

Later that year I was fortunate to meet Elisabeth Kübler-Ross, a young psychiatrist on the faculty who had developed an interest and expertise in death. She has since written widely and is recognized as an authority in the often ignored area of the dying patient. She conducted regular, optional seminars for students, house staff, nurses, and faculty on questions of death and dying. Her sessions were packed by medical workers eager to probe an area of daily concern that, most often, had been omitted from their education. The strongest point she left me with and, likely, a point that would have helped me deal with my stunning emotions of that surgical night was that impending death and death itself affects not only the patient and his family but everyone working with the patient. Many a person dies a hospital death bereft of conversations he or she would have liked to have had. The tendency of doctors on rounds, for instance, is to make light of the problems of a patient with a terminal illness. "How are you feeling today, Mr. Jones? You're looking good. Beautiful flowers. We'll see you tomorrow . . ." On the one level this makes sense. The physicians are attempting to keep Mr. Jones's spirits up by not dwelling on the obviously morbid side of his condition. On another level, the medical team is protecting itself. Dealing with death, as it is so often obliged to, it tries not to become mired in it. But the levity and flippancy of this approach denies Mr. Jones the opportunity to ask the questions that are surely in his mind. While the answers to his questions would not be easy, they might well afford him a measure of understanding and peace that he deserves. Instead he finds himself in the position of smiling and acting brave so as not to inconvenience or offend the doctors—a silly and inverted position by any standards.

Clearly there was not much time to talk to my surgical patient about his death. Yet I think I would have felt less loss after the experience had I had the benefit of Dr. Ross's provocative and extraordinary thinking prior to my night at the operating table. Death weighs heavily on anyone honest enough to stop and think about it. That realization is the beginning of the process of coping with rather than avoiding the phenomenon of death.

Sex as well as death is a topic that is poorly treated in medical school. The average physician, frequently the first one consulted on sexual problems, receives very little education that qualifies him to deal with the issues that will surely be posed in practice. My experience was no exception. Outside of a chance problem or two raised in my brief gynecology clerkship and a patient whom I encountered in out-patient psychiatry, my training was void of any discussion of sexual topics. This is by no means a new criticism and in recent years many medical schools have begun to provide courses in sex and sex education. But there is an issue that goes beyond the basic teaching of human sexuality that remains, to my knowledge, untouched by medical education; that is the sexuality of the physician himself.

(Because I use the word "himself," I by no means intend to imply that all doctors are men nor do I mean to limit the issue of sexuality to male doctors. On the contrary, I am sure that many of the problems I will touch on exist for female physicians. I use the male pronoun both for reasons of simplicity and because I am usually referring to myself and my own experience.)

"The woman probably has a cystocele," the urologist told me. "Her complaint is stress incontinence. Do you know what this means, Mullan?" I nodded vaguely, searching my memory. The urologist perceived my uncertainty. "A cystocele is a weakening of the wall of the vagina so that the bladder pushes down into it. Stress incontinence is the loss of urine with any stress—laughing, coughing, straining due to the weakening of the outflow channel—as in a cystocele. Go take a complete history, Mullan, do a complete physical and report back to me." His approach was surgical in the extreme and I obeyed.

I walked down the long hall of the Urology Clinic, passing many small examining rooms where patients dressed in street clothes waited for doctors. The hall was populated by a panoply of surgical gadgetry, autoclaves, microscopes, and the like. At the end I reached the room to which I had been dispatched. I pulled out of the pocket on the door the sheaf of papers that listed the height, weight, temperature, and address of my new patient and walked in.

Sitting alone in the cubicle was a stunning woman several years my junior. She smiled. I haltingly introduced myself and sat down at the small desk next to her. Her looks and manner stood in staggering juxtaposition to the mechanical manner in which I had just been introduced to her problem by the urologist. Some time had passed since I took that first laborious history from the vegetarian violinist and I no longer felt compelled to carry the clipboard around with me with all the questions outlined. Nonetheless, I found myself at a loss as to where to begin my cross examination of the young woman sitting near me wearing a thin blouse and a dapper, short skirt.

She rescued me. "Now I don't know whether you know what my problem is or not, Doctor Mullan, but for the last six months or so I have been losing urine into my underpants all the time. It happens most when I laugh. It doesn't matter if my bladder is full or empty. It still happens. That's kind of a silly problem for a grown girl like me so I thought I had better come and check it out." She was talking to my white coat. I was the doctor and, reasonably enough, she was treating me as such and presenting her trouble honestly and forthrightly. This time I didn't feel like a green student masquerading as doctor so much as I felt like a man, a sexual male incidentally dressed in a white coat.

Her straightforwardness helped orient me and focus my attention on the chore of history-taking. I proceeded efficiently enough to explore her present problem and review her past medical history. My attraction to her, I found, when kept in perspective, actually assisted me in getting to know her and in developing her problem. Simply put, I was interested in her and this pushed me to do a good job.

Examining her physically proved more troublesome again. This was the first time I was called on as a physician to physically explore a young, attractive woman. The experience caused conflict rather than sexual feeling. I examined her in rote fashion while hormonal cacophony reigned in my mind. I was so muddled by the time I investigated the site of my patient's trouble that I recorded almost nothing in my mind and could describe none of the physical findings to the urologist when I reported to him a few minutes later. He repeated the exam, discovered the cystocele, and scheduled her for surgery. She was admitted to the hospital at some later date and her problem, presumably, was cured. I doubt she sensed my anguish and I'm sure she wouldn't remember it or me. But I have not forgotten her or the conflict she first exposed me to.

Some months later Mary Sue White sat across from me in the small psychiatry office for twelve, perhaps fifteen, afternoons. She was my patient during my senior year out-patient psychiatry training. We met once a week for an hour during the training period. Once a month I met with a supervising psychiatrist to review our progress.

Mary Sue's case appeared clear enough. She was a twenty-one-year-old black woman with two children, and was going through a divorce. "This young woman is slightly depressed and anxious," read my introductory report, "and she needs some support during this difficult time in her life situation. With her young family, she is suffering some unresolved conflicts of adolescence. This needs work, too." Our first sessions moved along well. Bright and articulate, she was a handsome woman who quit her senior year of high school to give birth to the first of her two sons. She married her husband, Dwight, a week after her seventeenth birthday and, at twenty-one, found herself bored and frustrated. Dwight held down a regular job as a parking-lot attendant, liked movies, TV, beer, and the kids in that order. Over the previous year their marriage had degenerated into a running quarrel about everything. At last she demanded a divorce. Dwight still lived in the house but they both had lawyers and Mary Sue had a fledgling psychiatrist.

At our fourth or fifth visit she began to talk about her sexual problems. Even though sex was an everyday occurrence before and during their marriage, it never satisfied her. According to Mary Sue she hadn't realized she was missing anything until after the birth of her second child when she had some heart-to-heart talks with a friend. It seemed the friend had orgasm and Mary Sue became convinced she did not. She then discovered masturbation and found she could have orgasm by herself but still not with Dwight. Her frustration and anger grew. She told Dwight about the problem and he tried a little harder but nothing changed. The fights became worse and when I first met her she had decided that divorce was the only way out. Dwight, apparently, was whipped along on the end of her string. Reportedly he was willing to do whatever she wanted—divorce or no divorce. There were some flirtations in her life but no other men and no other real options. The only man she had ever had was Dwight. Despite her protests, I felt that she was deeply tied to her husband. Her questioning of sex stood as a query to herself, to her own ambition, to her own potential.

My abstractions concerning her problem (of which my tutor approved fully) were shattered in our sixth visit when she began describing the sexual dreams she had had about me. I stood out in contrast to Dwight, she explained, because I was doing something with my life and my education. Furthermore, I was gentle and understanding. After all, she asked, hadn't our whole relationship proved that? I had spent more time listening to her and worrying about her in six weeks than Dwight had in a whole marriage.

I was a set-up. This was transference, I said to myself in my cooler moments, but Freud could never have meant it like this. As our sessions progressed she reported that she used to masturbate thinking about me and that orgasm came more easily than ever. It was with an image of me in her mind that she could understand marriage and it was by thinking of me that she got through these depressing days. That completed the abstraction. I was to give her orgasm and complete her life, realize her ambitions, sate her appetite.

Although at base I doubted her real intent or ability to carry out what she proposed, her constant adulation and invitation upset me. While I understood the bind she led me toward, both her simple sexual appeal to me as a man and the recurrent *macho* notion that my sex might actually cure her led my thinking in an erotic direction. My tutor, with whom I finally sat down after three weeks of tortured sessions with Mary Sue, treated the problem brusquely. Sexual transference, he stated icily, is a frequent occurrence in psychotherapy and acting on it in any way is inappropriate and destructive. I had been read the chapter and verse. He admonished me to concentrate on things other than sex that disturbed her in her relationship with her husband. He neither asked nor seemed to perceive what I felt.

I stumblingly followed his advice although I never leveled with him again about my feelings. Mary Sue and I did explore other aspects of her relationship and life. But the invitation for sex always ran just beneath the surface of our conversations. At the end of one session when she related more sexual dreams to me, I stood and held her in my arms. It was a whimsical, erotic, anti-climactic moment. She was thrilled to be held and, in a sense, to have fulfilled her dreams. But she quickly pushed free of me and began to cry heartily. Her tears came from joy and disappointment. At once, she felt warmth and acceptance, guilt and fear. She was, after all, still married and Dwight was her husband. When she left the office a few minutes later she said she felt good and I believed her. She had tested herself and she knew where she stood. Already the experience had become a pleasurable memory for her. I, too, knew where I stood and was thankful for that.

Our remaining sessions were good ones devoid of sexual invocation or innuendo. We discussed at length what she could do to make her life and her marriage more satisfying. Significantly, she decided, with Dwight's support, to go back to school to get her high school equivalency degree before, perhaps, going on to college. When we parted we shook hands.

For some time I thought the sexual feelings I felt in relation to patients was a foible of my own that I would have to deal with in some way or other. It was, as I have mentioned, a topic never treated in medical school or thereafter. From talking with and observing classmates and other physicians I know it is a regular and, I think, understandable occurrence. Yet it is an area of medical taboo.

The attraction I felt as a man to an appealing woman stands not only as learned, societally determined behavior, but to some degree as instinctive behavior—my own sexuality. A sense of sex is part of all of us at all times. Wearing a white coat exempts no one. The job, and it is a tough one, is to put our sexuality into perspective so that it is destructive to neither the patient nor ourselves. For me medical school provided no teaching and no guidance in this difficult area. Physician sexuality remains a lonely topic in medicine. Professionalism and ethics, as they are traditionally known, as well as the alleged austerity of the white coat itself, dictate against even the discussion of the subject. The mere recognition of the issue threatens the assumed objectivity and sexless dispassion of the physician. About as dour and recriminatory a complaint as can be made by one physician about another is that "he messes with his patients." This attitude is both representative and supportive of the taboo that permeates the subject.

As with death, the obvious question that occurs is, can anything meaningful be taught about sexuality? Is it not clear that physicians must have the utmost ethical respect for the human body? What more need be said? Of course, the topic of sexuality would have to be handled quite differently from the average didactic subject. Seminars and group discussions could profitably focus on what "ethical respect for the human body" means or what hazards certain types of patients will pose for physicians. There is a rapidly expanding literature and cinema on the subject of human sexuality which could be used beneficially. The point of all this would not be to teach morality or mandate a code of behavior but to alert the physicians-to-be to a generic problem with which they will doubtless be involved. Discussion of human and physician sexuality would help to break the taboo and legitimize the subject so that doctors who suffer particular problems in the area could more easily seek guidance and support.

Sex, death, and life as well as fear and joy, pain and relief are the variable sinew of the human being and, hence, the fiber of medicine as well. That fiber came alive for me as a medical student. It was at once exciting and disturbing. It was a time for concentrating on people and diseases and not systems and policies. And yet I could not escape the presence of systems and policies lurking behind much of the disease and many of the people that I encountered. There was indeed a politics to much of what I saw—a politics that was not taught and rarely acknowledged. But it was there and it had much in common with what I had seen and felt in Mississippi. It was a politics that needed exposure and challenge.

3

Politics and Medicine

One Sunday morning in Mississippi, in the summer of 1965, I sat transfixed before a dim television set and watched Los Angeles in flames. I was dumbfounded. A place called Watts, a black ghetto I had never heard of, reeled under the impact of a self-imposed holocaust. The people of Watts had revolted and they were razing large sections of their neighborhood. I didn't understand it at all. I asked Cat and Mrs. Rust if they understood what was happening in Watts and they said they didn't. In my idealism, I couldn't conceive of the anger and hatred that could set an entire community on fire. The Civil Rights Movement was growing daily and it wouldn't be long, I thought, before places like Watts didn't exist anymore. Couldn't they see that? Why the need for violence?

Watts, of course, was only the beginning. It signaled revolt in the North and focused the attention of many Americans (me, for one) on the blight of countless urban neighborhoods. I came to realize that my platitudes, about how bad everything was in the South and, by contrast, how much more advanced we were in the North, were baseless. The ghettos of the northern cities were the flip side of the racist oppression I had seen in the South. To claim conscience and political concern but ignore the condition of millions of inner-city dwellers was ludicrous.

Chicago, for example, was not quiet. Racial tensions grew quickly in both black and white neighborhoods in Chicago in 1965 and 1966. The city, pointedly called the biggest town in Mississippi, braced itself fumblingly, hoping not to become another "riot" statistic. The Chicago scenario included the encrusted machine mayor, Richard J. Daley, a number of black politicians in Congress and the City Council, and small but numerous armies of street gangs and angry black youths. Into that mix came Martin Luther King, Jr. Moving his focus and the efforts of the Southern Christian Leadership Conference from the

South, Dr. King selected Chicago as the site of his first northern organizing drive.

The issue became housing integration. Southern in style and topical in content, integration of previously all-white neighborhoods had a significant appeal in black Chicago. With a burgeoning black middle class eager for housing outside of the ghettos and numerous white communities steeled against the arrival of any blacks at all, the relevance of a campaign aimed at racism in housing was clear. King moved quickly and well. Using black ghetto churches as a base and supported by a number of skillful lieutenants including Ralph Abernathy, Hosea Williams, and the youthful Jesse Jackson, King built a coalition of black activists and liberal whites. The strategy was exposure and non-violent confrontation and the vehicle was marches. Following the formula developed in the South, the Chicago Medical Committee for Human Rights was asked to provide medical support and coverage for the marches. "Medical Presence," as it came to be known, had been developing over the previous two years of southern confrontations. The essence of it was the presence of medical workers at marches or demonstrations where violence was possible. The role of the physicians, nurses, medical students, and so on, was twofold: first to provide emergency first aid for everything from blistered feet to gunshot wounds; and, second, to supply psychological support and encouragement for the demonstrators who might feel less apprehension about the confrontation knowing that there were medical people close at hand. For both reasons, MCHR volunteers wore identifying white coats or red-cross arm bands. Their supplies were toted in pockets, knapsacks, book bags, and purses.

Cicero, Gage Park, Chicago Lawn. Faceless neighborhoods on the outskirts of Chicago. Names known only as stops on the El map. Suddenly they were catchwords all over Chicago. Like Khe San or Iwo Jima, people spoke them with instant authority. And they were divisive words because no one used them without taking a side.

It was into these communities that Martin Luther King, Jr. ventured. Before each march we met excitedly, expectantly, at a church in a black community close to the target white neighborhood. The march leaders briefed us on the route, local hazards, and recent political developments. Then the singing began. They were the same songs we had sung in Holmes County, the same verses the Civil Rights Movement came to use all over the country. ("This little light of mine, I'm going to let it shine . . . All over Gage Park, I'm goin' let it shine . . .") Before we were finished King spoke. One or two staff members usually warmed us up, but King came on strong. Looking at the crowd somewhat absently as he did, gazing vaguely away to the side of the church, he would unexpectedly rivet his attention on you and drive home his point. Excitement rose within me as he spoke. His righteousness and his cunning, his intelligence and his charisma robbed me of the ability to resist his leadership. I was always far more ready to march after his sermons than before. He left me with no questions about the politics, correctness, or the timing of what we were about to do. Race in our own ranks never seemed to be an issue. We were disciplined, informed, and inspired foot soldiers when the meeting ended and we took to the march route after several verses of "We Shall Overcome."

I had not picketed a great deal before and it seemed strange to walk down the streets of a northern community and suffer more invective and hatred than I ever had in Mississippi. Stranger yet was the prevalence of the American Nazi Party at a number of the marches. Though painful, I could stand and, even, understand the fists and obscene gestures that we received. The inhabitants of the communities in which we marched saw us clearly as a threat. I could understand their being agitated and angry at our presence. But having the swastika thrust in my face block after block was an incomprehensible experience. Surely, for every Nazi present there was some man or woman standing in the crowd near him who had lost a father, brother, or son fighting the swastika. Yet race hate so gripped the populace that the symbol of Nazism did not trouble them. The enemy, they had decided, was in the street marching behind Martin Luther King. Little else mattered.

Surprisingly, very few people were injured during the marches. There were occasional scuffles and now and again someone threw something at us but, on balance, the crowds did very little physical damage. Often this was explained by the presence of large detachments of the Chicago Police Department. In some areas, such as Gage Park, the police walked two abreast, in tight formation on either side of the marchers. Although integrated, the Chicago police assigned very few black policemen to the marches. We speculated a good deal as to what the real feeling of the white cops was toward us. Were they not by race, style, and previous performance more a part of the crowd than they were part of the marchers? And how safe were we with members of the crowd guarding us from the crowd? The answer was not simple, because the uniformed white men with their baby-blue riot helmets did a good job of protecting us.

There was little for me to treat except sunburn and blisters. That was just as well since it meant that people weren't getting hurt and since I knew very little more first aid than I did when I was in Mississippi. Nonetheless, my presence at the march, strolling along with a black bag and a white coat, was important to the marchers and to me. The marches, in fact, took place at about the same time as I was being baptized by the Jewish Scientist, Mr. Gamoretz. The white coat, as I mentioned, had a special legitimizing influence on me in the context of the hospital. Wearing it at a political event had a different and new feeling, one that I liked. Wearing a white coat at a civil rights march symbolized to me the politicization of my medical experience. Mississippi made it appear to me that there were reasons I might want to be a doctor—there were people and causes for whom I would want to work. Gage Park and Cicero and the leadership of Martin Luther King brought that hope to life. I felt a slight guilt as I stole gauze pads and Ace bandages from the dressing cart in the treatment room on the surgical floor at the University of Chicago Hospital. But I knew where I was taking them and how I might have to use them. That knowledge made both the medical school and the march relevant.

About the time of the marches I moved to Woodlawn. Woodlawn is a black slum that abuts the university on its south side. With the aid of blockbusting real estate techniques and the post-war black migration north, Woodlawn, once a white neighborhood, rapidly became black in the fifties. The black influx had been contained or, better, defined by the Midway, a block-wide strip of park and parkway that cuts across the south side of the campus. To be sure, blacks lived to the north of the Midway mingling comfortably enough with the university community. But the Midway defined the difference between the poor and the very poor. Woodlawn became the home of the very poor with the attendant decay of housing, crime, graffiti, children, pimps, and rats. The university arched its back and dug in. Faced with the choice of abandoning the campus and fleeing to the suburbs or quarantining itself somehow, it elected to stay and construct an academic Maginot Line on the south side of the Midway. For a decade prior to the mid-sixties it had carefully and deliberately built a phalanx of stolid, functional, university buildings extending one block deep and ten or so blocks long between the approach of the slum and the tree-lined Midway. The Law School, the Social Work School, and the University Conference Center all rose between the Midway and Woodlawn. Looked at innocently, it made sense. The university needed to expand and the south side of the Midway was close at hand and available. Looked at in terms of real politics, it was the university's ostrich-like effort to survive in a changing urban scene it cared little to understand.

Few people from the university lived in Woodlawn. The line was clearly drawn in class, style, and color. There was in fact one large apartment building rented by the university one block deep into Woodlawn. Fondly called The Commune, it summoned to mind both images of the beleaguered Paris of 1870 (situated as it was) and the left political leanings of its occupants (a much-touted rumor). After that came the ghetto, untouched by the university, uninterested in the university, alive at all hours of the night or day, drab in any season of the year. Paved with broken glass, its streets were lined with dog shit, cigarette packages, bottle caps, milk cartons, rags, and pigeons. Room after room, house after house lit with 60-watt bulbs, Woodlawn was a raggedy and pale town within a city.

I moved to Woodlawn with Steve Cohen, a close friend and classmate. He too had ventured south to Mississippi in the summer of 1965 to work for MCHR. We found an apartment two blocks into Woodlawn and a short four blocks from the medical school. The building itself was in fairly good shape since our black landlord, Mr. Dobson, allowed no families with children. He was bent on protecting his investment until the arrival of a better day. "Kids destroy real estate," he told us. "That's all there is to it. So long as I can find people without kids I'm renting to them and keeping my place in one piece." We thought he might have second thoughts about renting to us since we were white. To the contrary, he was delighted we came along. First, we had no kids and second, we *were* white. Secretly, he confided to us, he had always thought his building was a good investment because it was so close to the university. Some day, he reasoned, the neighborhood would have to become integrated with university students and his real estate values would soar. He was sure we were the first wave and he welcomed us.

The building was the same vintage and architecture with the same hallway carpets and gray, painted wood back porches as countless apartments in Hyde Park, the university community, and many Chicago neighborhoods. Most of the buildings in Woodlawn, we learned in time, shared the same origin as the housing across the Midway and elsewhere in town. But the ghetto had changed it, overrun it. The carpets were gone. The hallway walls were crumbling. Gang battle slogans and the vernacular covered the outside walls. Windows were smashed, mailboxes ripped open or missing altogether, urine in vestibules, grass long since annihilated, doors bolted, destroyed, and reinforced again. Woodlawn had lost some time before, but it didn't matter. Landlords (Mr. Dobson being an exception) appeared only to collect the rent or had disappeared altogether despairing of their property.

Again the question occurred: was Woodlawn the product of the people, its inhabitants? Was it the victim of black procreativity and sloth? Or was it the product of the system, the American system, the Chicago system, the "largest town in Mississippi" system? We chose the latter conclusion. No one lived in Woodlawn because he wanted to, because it was the ideal community. The urine in the vestibules was as odious to others as it was to me. Folks in Woodlawn lived there because they had to. They suffered it because the life they led, the paths they followed, the system they were a part of offered little else. The road north out of Mississippi led inexorably to the John's Bargain Stores under the El, the bars on Sixty-third Street, the trammeled park with glass and bird droppings. For many the road went no further than Woodlawn. It was what America had to offer them and it consumed them. Sprawled on sheetless beds, the belt tourniquet barely free of their arms, crouched in alleys in the rain, or hunched over garbage fires in winter with their bottles in paper bags at their feet, or stiff-assing down Sixty-third Street with their skirts high on their thighs and a newly won ten-dollar bill in their bras, Woodlawn was *it* for many black people from the South.

Woodlawn became home for me and Steve. We looked, dressed, talked, and acted differently from almost everybody else in the community. Yet it felt comfortable in many ways. It shared much with Mississippi. We were again behind the lines and that felt good to us. There was much to be fought and much that needed change. We hoped to develop a block club to begin to discuss and resist some of the abuses that were rained on the neighborhood. We fantasized that our block club might be able to join hands with other such groups and begin to talk area-wide politics. We even saw the establishment of medical facilities or weekend clinics run by medical students and faculty from the medical school.

None of these things was destined to happen. We began talking block club to everyone we met shortly after we moved in. Some people thought we were political hacks, ward-heeler types. Others speculated that we were Communists, whatever they were. Some thought we were plain fools. A few listened to us, and came to the first meeting at our house. Twelve or fifteen people showed in all and sat nervously around half expecting a religious experience, half wanting an interracial orgy. Steve and I opened by stating honestly and simply why we were there. It was our hope, we said, to start a regular meeting group that could discuss the problems of the community and decide on a program to combat them. People happily talked about the many ills of the neighborhood. Some thought the police were too tough, some too lenient. Some thought the mayor was to blame for the litter in the streets, some thought the "trashy" people themselves. And so it went. While all recognized the same grievances, there was little agreement as to causes or remedies.

The block club met two or three times before it died. Unlike the organization in Mississippi, our block club had no base in the people. There was no Freedom Democratic party in Woodlawn, no Movement, no songs, and no heroes. There were just disorganized, often disheartened, people steeled as well as possible against the facts of Woodlawn life. Our ideals, our energy, even our previous experience meant little against the compelling reality of Woodlawn. Folks came to the block club meeting, talked about what they saw, saw no way to change it, and went on about their business. We remained friends with a number of the people who had come to the meetings but after a month or so we gave up on the ambitious organizational schemes and settled down to just live in Woodlawn.

We stayed more than two years in Mr. Dobson's building. Our apartment was comfortable and convenient. Shopping on Sixty-third Street, frequenting local merchants, walking the neighborhood both day and night, we got to know the community. It was a good experience and a revealing one but it was not always easy. I often felt self-conscious or nervous. At night especially I always expected trouble. Luckily, it never happened. Steve and I often fell victims to a certain gentle fleecing that was popular sport in the neighborhood. It frequently happened at dusk when one or the other of us was walking home alone. A group of teenagers would suddenly appear and be everywhere. "Hey, brother," one of them would say, "how about a quarter? I need a quarter awful bad." Thinking a quarter was not a bad deal for my liberty, I would try to comply. "Now, my friend here, he needs a quarter bad, too. Real bad." So it would go until I had forked up enough money to make everybody richer by twenty-five cents. They obligingly took paper money promising to make change and distribute it themselves. If I didn't have enough for a quarter all around, they agreeably took what I had and promised to look me up again. They were always businesslike and reasonable. I never tested their ire. Steve and I saw it as a tariff for living in the neighborhood. We told Mr. Dobson about the game and he was furious.

Life changed suddenly one day in the spring of 1968. A gaunt white man in Memphis, Tennessee shot and killed the ceremonial leader of the striking garbage men. Martin Luther King, Jr. was dead and the black communities of Chicago erupted in an agonized, holocaustic funeral ceremony. Steve and I didn't go home for three days, fearing that any white face on the street might provoke anger. When we did we discovered much looting and window smashing in the neighborhood but no burning. Our cat was hungry and angry but our apartment remained untouched. For a time we returned to the apartment during the day but slept elsewhere at night. After several weeks we again slept in the apartment, but always felt like stowaways in the night hoping no one would find us before dawn. Any romantic notions that we might have had about being exempted from the wrath of the community because we were "friendly" whites was smashed by any number of fist-shaking and name-calling incidents that occurred during these months. The city is not like the countryside where someone is known for himself. On the city streets you are a color, a sex, and a size. We were medium-sized white boys and those were not good credentials in Woodlawn in the spring of 1968. As it happened, medical school was drawing to a close for us. We packed our few belongings, gave our cat away, said good-by to the few friends we had in the community and to Mr. Dobson (who was finally convinced that we were not the real first wave) and left. We had observed a fetid, vibrant black American slum for two and a half years and, I think, personally benefited a great deal from the experience. But we left Woodlawn unchanged, untouched by our experience. We *were* two medium-sized white boys who probably had no business thinking we could enlighten or redirect somebody else's neighborhood with some idealism, a little Mississippi experience, and a few meetings. Woodlawn had hardly noticed us amid the general scramble.

"Dumb," the obstetrical resident assured us. "The colored women we deliver here are too dumb to have postpartum depressions. That's just plain fact." He was referring to the black women of the South Side of Chicago, many of whom came to the University of Chicago Hospital for obstetrical care. The students, heads bent, took careful notes as the resident continued his lecture.

Medical "facts" are rarely free of interpretation, innuendo, and value judgment. To describe the observed absence of depression after delivery in black women in Chicago as a product of "dumbness" is clearly a value judgment, a racist value judgment, on the part of the resident. Yet that very sort of comment, that fact *cum* prejudice, that thoughtless slur against an entire population occurred frequently in our medical teachings. The students, for the most part, accepted such commentary and integrated it into their own thinking. And why not? They had been taught to take notes, memorize, and repeat. That was medical education. Moreover, the denigrations were not aimed at them. The students were white, male, and, like the resident, comfortably removed from the target of his remarks—poor black women. The statement seemed plausible if harsh and, like many others, it passed unchallenged.

Our class was not built for challenge. Like all other medical school classes, we were chosen first and foremost on the grounds of academic ability as determined by traditional standards—college performance. That, of course, said a great deal about who we were, where we came from, and what kind of priorities we shared. First of all we had made it *to* college, usually a well-recognized and frequently an expensive college. Second, we had graduated from college in the upper ranks of our classes, suggesting a certain intelligence but also an acceptance of and a success within the system. Third, we had neither debts nor family commitments, illness nor hunger that drove us to translate our college achievement into immediate income. And finally, most of us had come from sufficiently affluent backgrounds so that we could foot the bill for tuition and four years of room and board with little or no income.

These are by no means bad criteria for selecting stable individuals with sufficient mental equipment to handle the rigors of a traditional medical curriculum. But they are criteria guaranteed to cull out a fairly uniform and narrow segment of American youth, one much like the generation before, and one not particularly equipped for challenge. Our class of 75, for example, was comprised of 68 white males, half a dozen women, and a lone black. The black came not from Chicago, not from Illinois, not from the United States, but from Nigeria. We had no Puerto Ricans, no Chicanos, no Appalachian whites, and, in fact, no one from any background of ethnically identifiable poverty.

We were overwhelmingly white men, young and ambitious, bent on careers in medicine as traditionally defined—research and private practice.

Our medical school class was not very different from others around the United States. Yet in spite of our uniformity and our apparent similarity to the classes that had been chosen and had graduated before us, an unlikely series of events began to occur at the University of Chicago and elsewhere. By the mid-1960s many medical students had started to question the role of medicine in American life. In part it was the times. Reexamination, objection, and protest were rapidly replacing political apathy and fraternity pranks as hallmarks of the student way of life. To a greater degree, though, it was medicine itself that called for reappraisal and reform. To many of us the American Medical Association symbolized medicine in America. Overfed and complacent, the "voice" of organized medicine seemed completely self-serving and ignorant of the health problems that beset many Americans. They had battled too long to block the involvement of the government in the care of its people. They had lobbied too hard to restrict the number of students in medical schools to keep physicians' prices high. On issue after issue the AMA supported the rich, the entrenched, and the reactionary.

Medical schools, of course, weren't the AMA; we understood that. In fact, medical school faculties generally have shunned organized medicine, leaving the county, state, and national organizations entirely in the hands of private practitioners. There is, therefore, a wide chasm between the teachers of medicine and the practitioners of medicine. And yet, undeniably, the schools of medicine produced the physicians of the nation who became the AMA in all its affluence and self-satisfied conservatism. If we could not argue that the medical schools of the country created the AMA, at least it was clear that they did nothing socially or educationally to prevent its development and good health. There had to be—and there was—a system functioning in and around schools of medicine that narrowly determined who would become physicians and what would be the limited bounds of their concern. That system invited analysis, exposure, and resistance.

In 1965 the Students for a Democratic Society (SDS) was five years old. Many medical students had been exposed to SDS as undergraduates. A number of us had been south working for MCHR, the Student Non-Violent Coordinating Committee (SNCC), or the Freedom Democratic party. The campuses of America's universities had awakened from their long slumber of the fifties and were experiencing a spate of organizational efforts. In medical school there had been little or no political activity since the death of a group called the Association of Interns and Medical Students (AIMS) in the early fifties. AIMS came into being in the late thirties and was borne aloft for more than a decade by the efforts of a group of energetic and socially aware medical students who fought for national health insurance, chest X-rays for all medical workers, and pay for interns, published a national journal, and held annual meetings. But in 1952 the American Medical Association published a picture of a student rally in Holland where two AIMS leaders were shown marching beside two alleged European Communists. The red scare was on and AIMS had little with which to fight. National advertising was quickly withdrawn from their journal, which could not support itself. Publication ceased, membership dwindled, and the organization foundered. The AMA responded with a "loan" of $50,000 to a group of students calling themselves the Student American Medical Association (SAMA). Between the early fifties and the mid-sixties SAMA existed alone, selling life insurance, sponsoring dances, and circulating a periodical filled with third-rate medical articles.

By 1965 we were ready for something more than SAMA. Our New Frontier liberalism, at the least, beckoned us to do something to make our medical education more relevant, more likely to produce a brand of doctor other than the AMA stereotype. Slowly at first, and spontaneously, a number of mild medical-campus student organizing efforts began to take shape. In Boston students worked in the Mission Hill Extension Housing Project to assist families in getting health care. Teams of students from San Francisco journeyed to Delano, California, to help the striking farm workers establish a medical service. In Chicago we began working with the Woodlawn Organization and the Chicago Council on Biomedical Careers to gain entry for blacks into health science schools. Initially there was no coordination and no exchange of information among the programs at various schools. Nonetheless, they had several key features in common. First, the content of the projects was always to some degree political and social. Second, the efforts were almost always extramural, carrying the students away from the traditional seat of medical education, the medical center, into the community. Third, often the programs crossed time-honored professional lines including nursing and dental students as well as medical students. Finally, and most important, the projects were always student initiated and student run. The institutions were not evolving and carrying their students with them. Rather, the students had changed and they were struggling to drag their schools along behind them.

Far and away the most significant student organizing effort took place in Los Angeles. There, with the leadership of two University of Southern California medical students, Bill Bronston and Mic McGarvey, a closely knit, city-wide health student organization called the Student Medical Conference (SMC) came to life. The USC students set the style and pace of the organization, raising funds for an impressive, student-run lecture series featuring nationally known figures and controversial topics such as abortion, war, and racism. They published a handsome magazine called *Borborygmi* (literally, stomach rumbles), a student journal that tackled questions of curriculum, politics, and medicine. Students from other area schools participated in community health projects in Los Angeles, trips to Delano in support of the farm workers, and legislative lobbying for a therapeutic abortion bill. Four Student Medical Conference members spent the summer of 1965 in Mississippi and Louisiana working with MCHR.

The Student Medical Conference was important not only for the vigor and sophistication of its program but for the breadth of its vision. The SMC and particularly its colorful leader, Bill Bronston, saw the Los Angeles program as a precursor and a format for health science student organizing all over the country. In the spring of 1965 Bronston, then finishing his senior year at medical school, set about spreading the news of the SMC around the country. Descendant of a European revolutionary, son of a Hollywood producer, and husband of a TWA stewardess (which allowed him to fly at reduced rates), Bronston set off cross-country to find and meet with health science students interested in change. The fact of the existence of the SMC, as well as its obvious success, he reasoned, would serve to catalyze and focus the scattered and as yet uncoordinated student concern with the political and social state of health in America. Charismatic, articulate, and, to some, threatening, Bronston sparked enthusiasm and controversy wherever he touched down. His message was clear and generally well received; health student action programs were feasible, politically crucial, and educationally mandatory if the priorities and allegiances of American medicine were to change at all.

In Chicago his effect was powerful. Several of us at the University of Chicago had spent the year grumbling about the state of our education and hoping we could entice a lecturer or two to discuss medical ethics or medical politics with us. MCHR leaders Quentin Young and Irene Turner gathered six or eight of us together to meet Bronston when he came to Chicago. It was final exam week and rounding us up was not easy. Suddenly Bronston was describing and detailing things we had only dreamed about. Bearded and intense, he held us spellbound. For each point he made, for every project he described he produced flyers, posters, and newspapers to illustrate the program. *Borborygmi* was artistically beautiful and politically strong. We had never seen a student medical journal except SAMA's *The New Physician,* which published nothing of specific interest to the student and filled its pages with scientific articles which had been turned down elsewhere. *Borborygmi* talked about the curriculum, ethics, students in the ghetto, and students in the grape vineyards. While we had mused about the possibility of student-sponsored lectures they had carried out a forum series that would have made most theatrical agents jealous. While we had speculated about students in the community they had put dozens to work around Los Angeles and in the San Joaquin Valley. The SMC had an impressive program and Bronston was a superb salesman.

Those of us who spent the evening with Bronston were sold. We agreed to organize an interscholastic, interdisciplinary health student group devoted to curricular reform and community service in Chicago. More important, we agreed to host a national student convention in the fall of 1965. Sixty-five students from twenty-five schools of medicine, nursing, and dentistry around the country came to that meeting, the grist of which proved to be the sharing of information. No one had any idea of the scope of student unrest and innovation. If the get-together had adjourned after the exchange of reports from the various schools it would have been worthwhile. More than that, however, there was a sense of kinship and commonality from the outset. The diagnoses as well as the treatments tried by students from different cities and different disciplines were strikingly similar. Irrelevance, the absence of humanism, political conservatism, and the failure to recognize or deal with blatant social problems were the frequent complaints. Extramural action programs, student lecture series, and student publications were the common responses. The group was more than an activist SAMA. Almost a third of the students were in nursing or dentistry and we all accepted the axiom that medicine had to overcome the destructive barriers placed between the several specialties within health science. Any organization devoted to that change had to be interdisciplinary itself. After much debate we decided to call ourselves the Student Health Organization (SHO) to emphasize that we were not merely a *medical* society. Fashioned consciously after the World Health Organization, we announced in our statement of purposes that in our view "Health was total physical, mental, and social well-being and not merely the absence of disease."

Bronston arranged to have Paul Dudley White fly to Chicago to address the gathering. The renowned and aging cardiologist, known for his progressive views on the organization and practice of medicine, willingly took his weekend to join our small group of future nurses, dentists, and doctors. His message, though, proved perplexing and one I have since thought about frequently. What we were doing, he said, was commendable, necessary, topical. Had he been our age, he assured us, he would have been with us. Then, however, he launched into a nostalgic and, no doubt, accurate account of his own career. Medical school was his most important moment and he dwelled on it at length. He had graduated second in his class from Harvard, which started him on an impressive academic career that saw him eventually founding the specialty of cardiology. It was his good start, graduating second in his class at Harvard, he told us time and again, that assured him the position he achieved later in life. Then, once he was prominent and widely respected, he let his political views be known. With degrees and publications and accolades behind him, he began his political and social proselytizing. This, he insisted, was the way to do it.

As I listened to him, I reflected on the fact that the following day at nine in the morning I had my first pathology exam of the new academic year. I knew well that three-quarters of my class were studying hard for the test even as I sat there listening to Dr. White. My involvement in SHO promised to detract from my conventional work in a way that would guarantee that I would graduate nowhere near number two in the class. In fact, the stance of the student activist was precisely contrary to what the elderly physician preached. We were opting to interrupt our educations and our professions immediately and take issue with what we felt was wrong. I did and I do respect what Dr. White achieved medically and socially in his long career. But some time after hearing him speak I concluded that he was wrong. Many young people have criticisms of the systems in which they grow up. For a variety of reasons they mute their objections and accomplish their educational goals, believing all the time that they will at some more powerful time in the future speak up and argue for change. But, one way or another, the time never comes. The process itself changes the student, the novitiate, the youth, the learner. We all become apologists for the systems that produce us. It is a rare and exceptionally strong individual who can lie low through a long training and conditioning process and at the end speak out with anything resembling the virgin anger that he might have voiced early on. I am willing to accept that Paul Dudley White was an exception to this, but he is the rare instance. The SHO was founded on the premise that to feel indignation and speak, to sense wrong and to criticize, to see oppression and to act was good. In his own way Dr. White helped focus that thought in many of our minds.

For me that first SHO meeting was fabulously exciting. Most of the people there were new to me, but their attitudes, their aspirations, and their complaints were uncannily familiar—they were mine. Seated in their midst I was no longer a misfit, a malcontent, as I so often had felt since arriving at medical school. Like them I had become a foot soldier in a new army—a guerrilla brigade preparing to disperse again to do battle singly or in small units against apathy, irrelevance, and conservatism in our education and our lives.

I remember thinking, while taking the pathology exam the following morning that I might not do well on the test, but there was a good reason for my mediocre performance—a reason that several dozen new friends in New York and Los Angeles, in Boston and San Francisco would understand. There was solace in knowing that they also labored for divided and sometimes contrary masters, their schooling and their principles.

In the fall of 1965 and the winter of 1966 the SHO of Chicago came to life. Waller, beard intact, classmate Lambert King, and a handful of University of Chicago students along with representatives from ten or so Chicago area medical, nursing, and social work schools drew up a charter and set about an interscholastic appraisal of our educations. Terry Fonville, medical student at the University of Illinois, developed and edited *YES*, the journal of the SHO of Chicago. *YES* symbolized the positivism and the commitment of the organization. Fonville quoted Baldwin on the front cover of the first issue and Joyce on the back. "This is why one must say Yes to life," wrote the former, "and embrace it wherever it is found—and it is found in terrible places; nevertheless, there it is; and if the father can say, Yes, Lord, the child can learn that most difficult of words, Amen." And Joyce added,

". . . and then I asked him with my eyes to ask again yes and then he asked me would I yes to say yes my mountain flower and first I put my arms around him yes and drew him down to me so he could feel my breasts all perfume yes and his heart was going like mad and yes I said yes I will Yes."

YES grew up in the tradition of *Borborygmi*, the original USC publication. Humanism and politics were its twin themes as they related to the practice of medicine in the United States. Every issue contained art work, photography, and poetry as well as essays and reports on the activities of the organization on the various campuses. The artistic commentary in *YES* was neatly tied to the medical and political efforts of the SHO and contrasted eloquently with the artless and frequently thoughtless content of the average health science school course offering. We distributed hundreds of copies of each issue to medical and nursing students throughout Chicago.

YES was only one of a number of SHO publications that began to appear around the country. The most significant was *Encounter* which took over from *Borborygmi* in 1966 and apeared four or five times a year through 1969 as the national journal of the SHO. More than any single element (except perhaps friendship) *Encounter* was responsible for the cogent and articulate development of the SHO as a national movement. *Encounter*'s Los Angeles based editors filled its pages with the best student writing from around the country. Throughout its articles there ran a constant challenge to the student readership to change the face of American medicine. Sometimes the criticism was ironic, such as the automobile ad reproduced from the *AMA News* without comment:

b. Columbus, O.	1922
B.S.	1943
M.D.	1947
Amer. Coll. Surgs.	1953
Asst, prof. surgery	1956
Assoc. prof. surgery	1959
Private practice, Chi.	1963
CADILLAC	1967

At other times it was blunt, as in a quotation from Voltaire on doctors: "Men who prescribe medicine of which they know little, to cure diseases of which they know less, in human beings of whom they know nothing."

The activities and the results of SHO agitation varied from campus to campus. At the University of Chicago, for instance, we were successful in establishing a student-run lecture series that we called the Student Medical Forum after its Los Angeles counterpart. The university and the faculty gave us moral and financial backing as we invited speakers on ghetto medicine, osteopathy, abortion, government health care, and the future of medicine. Our quests included the late Saul Alinsky, Robert Coles, Barry Commoner, Jack Geiger, and the itinerant organizer himself, Bill Bronston. Elsewhere educational reform including student involvement on medical school curriculum, admissions, and promotions committees became the focus of SHO activity. The most important single development for the SHO during this period was the advent of Summer Projects. Building on the SHO principle of extramural community service projects, the SMC succeeded in obtaining a $200,000 grant from the Office of Economic Opportunity to put one hundred medical, nursing, and dental students to work in impoverished areas of California during the summer of 1966. They had no difficulty obtaining the recruits who helped organize clinics for migrants, did dental screening in Watts, worked out of private physicians' offices in poor counties designing better methods of patient-screening and coverage, and the like. While the students clearly didn't restructure medical care in California they did perform valuable community service jobs, many of which bore results long after they returned to school. Both the students and the preceptors (usually physicians or nurses) who worked with them felt that the education the summer workers received in the health care system was unequaled in medical curricula anywhere. Most important for the SHO, the Summer Project proved a training ground for future SHO leaders around the country. Almost half the students who worked in California in the summer of 1966 were from schools in other parts of the country. Returning as they did to their campuses in the fall they were ready to organize their colleagues and begin talking about Summer Projects of their own.

In the summer of 1967 the SHO sponsored three Summer Projects —in New York, in Chicago, and again in California. Funds for the programs came from several federal agencies including the OEO. I worked on developing and coordinating the Chicago project and when it was over several things were clear to me. First, working as they did on the streets of Chicago well outside the medical centers, the students saw medical and social problems from a very different vantage point than they would at any other time in their educations. They fought a thousand battles—with a drugstore to get tongue blades for a street clinic; with a medical center to accept their referrals; with the mayor to get paid; with a street gang to keep from being annihilated. Second, they got to know each other, students generally somewhat different from their classmates, in varied disciplines, from many parts of the country, most often critical of the medical and medical school status quo. Many of the bonds—personal and medical—developed on the SHO projects in Chicago and elsewhere outlasted the SHO itself and have remained important in the growth of new attitudes among health workers.

The Student Health Projects of these years and, indeed, the SHO itself, were conceived in a spirit of temperate protest. Most of us still believed that the Democratic liberals in Washington (who, after all, supported our program generously) had the capability of building a better and a more democratic nation. Our criticisms were based primarily on simple idealism. We felt, for instance, that our schools weren't doing their part in the ghettos that so often surrounded them. Yet rarely did we discuss the financial or social roots of the universities and what bearing they might have on the neglect we catalogued. Not until several years later did we pay much attention to the aggressive roles that many universities played in the destruction or engulfment of contiguous neighborhoods. Outside of our schools we tended to confine our debate and criticism to the medical system itself, rarely looking beyond to the economic practices and social policies that, in fact, predetermined the medical reality.

Yet, as we became more involved in the problems of the poor and the politics of medicine and medical schools, our beliefs began to change. Almost imperceptibly at first we drifted away from the New Frontier notions that had launched us into politics. What we were experiencing did not square well with the simple idealism of earlier years. We were beginning to sense an interconnection between the events we observed, a consistency behind American politics that suggested a system rather than mere oversight or accident. As we began to connect our observations about the ghettos, medical schools, and medical care, as we started to discuss and analyze a system rather than an isolated series of observations, we left the New Frontier and became a part of the growing New Left. As such we saw ourselves as a new and independent development, linked to our student peers but rooted in no previous part of the American experience. We had no formal

Communists in our ranks. Generally we knew nothing of labor history or class theory. Dylan was more a hero than Che and no one had ever heard of Gus Hall.

In the years following 1965 the war became an increasingly important subject. Many students involved in SHO became active in the anti-war movement, giving time and money to organizing, draft counseling, and demonstrations. Many of us, though, felt the war and SHO should be kept separate. The SHO, we argued, had a job to do in the arena of health science and, while we were against the war, we shouldn't drag it into the SHO, risking the alienation of prestigious supporters and federal funding. I personally argued this position consistently for several years. I argued it fervently and, I now think, wrongly.

In the end it didn't matter because the war was relentless and inescapable. At the outset we could avoid it or at least isolate it as a topic, a pestilence, to be treated separately. But that could not last because the war permeated our lives as well as our consciences. The male students in the SHO all faced the draft upon completion of their training. For a time there was even a serious proposition that nurses should be subject to the draft. Medical personnel forfeited virtually all deferments. Neither age nor family status, neither flat feet nor myopia could stave off the ultimate likelihood of our being sent to Viet Nam to take part in a war we opposed. The question of the war became less academic and more real for us with each passing month.

Since SHO groups around the country were reluctant to tackle the war directly, a movement was started outside of the SHO to enlist medical student resistance to the Vietnamese conflict. The "Pledge of Non-Participation," as it came to be known, started on the West Coast and traveled the country gaining some five hundred signatures of commitment during the period from 1967 to 1969. "In the name of freedom," it read, "the United States is waging an unjustifiable war in Viet Nam and is causing incalculable suffering. It is the goal of the medical profession to prevent and relieve human suffering. My effort to pursue this goal is meaningless in the context of this war. Therefore, I refuse to serve in the armed forces in Viet Nam; so that I may exercise my profession with conscience and dignity I intend to seek means to serve my country and humanity which are compatible with the preservation and enrichment of life." The statement bound no one to a set course of action. Broad enough to attract pacifists and militants, it invited support from all students opposed to the war.

Yet I found it hard to sign, and once having committed myself to the pledge, I discovered signatures were never easy to collect. Not only did the pledge require a moral or political belief that the war was unjust but it asked the individual's signature in testimony to that conviction. No one knew what the signature might mean. We were increasingly aware of government surveillance and it seemed unlikely that a freely circulating list of medical students committed not to serve in the military in Viet Nam would long escape the Selective Service, the FBI, and the Pentagon. Would such information preclude our serving in the military in any capacity or would we be obliged to serve as enlisted men, as left-wing physicians had been forced to do in the fifties? Would it damage Conscientious Objector applications? Would it be prime evidence against us in some new McCarthyite pogrom? Would it, in the end, matter?

The battle never materialized. Most likely the fact that we were signatories of the pledge resides somewhere in the government's files. Perhaps the information is fodder for some future skirmish, but probably not. Nonetheless, in contrast to what I felt at the time, the pledge and our signatures had a meaning despite the absence of confrontation with the government. Our signatures stood as an act of resistance. "My effort to pursue that goal is meaningless . . . ," we stated, "Therefore, I refuse to serve . . ." For most of us the push never came to shove and we served a quiet two years in the Public Health Service, entered the military but avoided Viet Nam, or secured Conscientious Objector status. But the statement of conscience signed willingly by hundreds of future physicians placing themselves in potential legal and, perhaps, physical resistance to their government stands as a significant moral and political act. Moreover, the students did not challenge the government out of any sense of individual desperation or personal gain. The easiest route, far and away, was compliance. Doctors were not dying in Viet Nam. The usual tour abroad—if indeed one actually went to Southeast Asia—was a year. Residency, practice, and the good life waited beyond. The signature promised only trouble. In a sense it made us outlaws. It was proof that our objection had gone beyond simple talk and had taken us to a point where we might have to pay for our beliefs with our comfort or well-being. That act took us beyond liberalism once and for all and made us a more solid part of the New Left. Our politics had become activist. No longer did we believe that someone else, some well-intentioned politician or administrator, would change things. If change was to occur, if the war was to be stopped, we and people like us would have to risk ourselves. That mentality, the mentality with which we signed, embodied a new politics, one significantly different from the moderate liberalism with which I had come to political adulthood.

Something else happened to my own thinking about the war during this period. Growing up in the America of the 1950s, remembering vaguely the tone and tenor of Joe McCarthy, rooting passionately as I had for the good guys against the "faceless Chinese hordes" in the Korean War, it was not easy to approach the National Liberation Front and the North Vietnamese with much objectivity. My first objections to the war came simply enough out of a sense of indignation. It seemed wrong for the 500,000 Americans with M-16s and napalm to be running amuck in a tiny nation of rice paddies and water buffalo. It abused my sense of fair play. The principles allegedly being fought for hardly seemed as supportable or demonstrable as the principles that were obviously being violated. Somewhere along the line my thinking changed. I began to realize that what the generals had in South Viet Nam was, indeed, much like what we had in this country. Exploitation and self-aggrandizement were king. A person was what he could buy—including pieces of the government. South Viet Nam was a crude, impoverished caricature of the United States. The North, by contrast, seemed to be gamely, bravely trying to break that cycle of exploitation. Their values, their medical system, their respect for women, their provision of a basic standard of living for all their citizens seemed much closer to my own sense of justice than anything South Viet Nam was or pretended to be. In revolt against my upbringing and in spite of my knowledge that Americans were fighting and dying, I found myself not simply against the war but, rather, *for* the North Vietnamese and the NLF.

As hard as I argued against the involvement of the SHO in the anti-war movement in early years, the same process that assaulted and changed my thinking captured the organization as a whole. Our liberal cocoon was ill-fated. As we became more outspoken in our resistance to the war, we did alienate many professors, deans, and benefactors. More important, we discouraged or confused many of our fellow students. While the war was a motivating and binding issue for some of us, it proved a schismatic and rending subject in general. When we challenged medical education and health care for the poor we received a sympathetic or, at the least, bemused hearing from students and faculty alike. When we stood up against the war, many responded with anger or disdain. We had passed from the safe realm of liberal idealism to the domain of radical politics and the constituency, the tactics, and the stakes were different.

By 1968 the Student Health Organization had reached its high point as a national movement. No formal national organization existed but the shared philosophy and the parallel programs of the many local and regional groups added up to a strong and cohesive national confederation. The national meeting held in February of 1968 in Detroit attracted almost four hundred health science students all of whom raised the money for their own travel expenses. The name of the meeting (like all others of a national character) was carefully pluralized—the Assembly of the Student Health Organizations. That summer six hundred health science students worked on Student Health Projects in nine areas. And yet the SHO faced a grave crisis. The potential clearly existed in 1968 to establish the SHO as a formal national organization with offices, officers, full-time staff, travel funds, and improved communications. Certainly we had a large enough and broad enough constituency and the demonstrated ability to raise funds—both important prerequisites to forming a national structure. Many SHO members, though, questioned the wisdom of building a national hierarchy that might stifle local growth and/or be subverted by personal ambition or government espionage. At the Detroit convention a hot debate took place on the merits of national versus local emphasis with the clear edge going to a local preference. Increasing numbers of SHO members had come to distrust national political leaders and felt they had ample evidence of the abuse of power in Washington. They had little reason to believe that their peers would do any better if allowed to accumulate power and prestige as national health student leaders. The revelation that the government had spied on and, in some instances, bought political parties, labor unions, and even the National Student Association was fresh in everybody's mind. What was to exempt the SHO from such a fate?

Then too, there was the question of organizational philosophy and direction. Between Bronston's first salvos in 1964 and the massive Detroit meeting of 1968, the SHO had grown and functioned without a formal constitution. It is perhaps a testimony to the obviousness of the need for reform in health science schools that we worked for as long and as well as we did without more precise organizational ground rules. But by 1968 the adherents of the SHO had many differing ideas about what the organization should be. The role of the SHO as an anti-war organization was clearly the question that divided people most sharply. The continued acceptance of government money also proved an issue of contention, as did the establishment of a national office, relations with other organizations, and a number of lesser questions. Writing in *YES*, Henry Kahn, a Harvard medical student who had been active in the SHO from the start, put the problem well:

[The SHO] is sort of like a tremendous psychedelic bus cruising to pick up the guys who ought to make this trip. Now each of us has to propose a place to go. It's not enough only to be on the bus, or even to have packed it to capacity. Any capable bureaucrat might have performed that trick. This is the juncture that calls for leadership, for ideas. . . . Here then is where we have to talk seriously about programmatic goals and content. We should have given this more consideration back when we were busy rounding up passengers. . . . The bus is filled now and we find that the ticket-master is only willing to suggest the same old road. Things are jumping too fast, even among health science students, for this situation to be tolerated long. In my view, the bus had better start zipping down some significantly new, perhaps uncharted highway, or it will soon find itself overloaded and stuck.

Things *were* jumping fast. In student politics in general, and in health student politics in particular, a kind of freneticism reigned. Month by month, week by week issues changed, new rhetoric appeared, new organizations formed and faded. The Yippies hit the scene; the Weathermen, the Weather People and, eventually, the Weather Underground joined the American body politic. The Chicago Convention happened. The Black Panthers arose and the Young Lords and, later, the White Panthers. And behind it all, fueling or, at least focusing much of it, the war ground on.

Among students and among political radicals, trust was at low ebb. That fact as much as anything discouraged the creation of large organizations and promoted the formation of collectives—small groups of like-minded people living and working together. There were many arguments for the collective approach to life but above all it insured an intimacy and a trust of those one worked with.

The SHO, of course, already had a built-in mini-structure—the local organizations. They were not collectives in the strict sense of the word but they were small groupings of people who knew and trusted one another. In spite of the potential—some argued, necessity—for a national organization, the Assembly of the Student Health Organizations essentially vetoed the notion at the Detroit meeting. The decision was made to minimize national organizational activity and encourage local programs, recruitment, and fund raising. The rationale was that local groups could democratically decide the sticky issues about war policy, government grants, and the like without being dictated to by some national body. Moreover, local people could monitor their fellows and, it was hoped, prevent government snooping, subversion, and payoffs.

That approach, decided on at the height of SHO power, proved a reasonable but a suicidal one. The corollary of a weak national focus in 1968 was the rapid diffusion of direction and identity for the movement as a whole. Partially because some changes had been achieved in health science schools and partially because lecture series and summer projects seemed inconsequential in the face of the war and the state of the nation, educational reform ceased to be a unifying issue for the SHO. Stripped of that point of philosophical accord, lacking a constitution, adrift in the stormy political waters of the late 1960s, the SHO fell apart. Some groups continued to carry out important and successful local programs for several more years but the national focus, the camaraderie that Bronston had brought to life, died. Perhaps the SHO would have crumbled or splintered even with a strong national structure; certainly few organizations spawned by the politics of the sixties survived the turmoil of the late sixties and the trial of the war. But without a binding structure, local SHO groups "zipped" along in a dozen different directions.

The 1969 National Assembly held in Philadelphia still attracted several hundred participants but it lacked leadership, common direction, or the ability to commit anybody to anything. It was an organizational death agony. Anti-war militants, demands for minority admissions to medical schools, women's power, and a guerrilla theater all captured the agenda for a time. Nobody and no program held the causes together and people left disgruntled for as many reasons as there were issues. It was the last SHO convention.

A national office of sorts, started in 1968 with a Carnegie Corporation grant, limped along until 1970. It enjoyed no authority of any sort and was called the SHO Service Center to emphasize its purely supportive nature. I attended a meeting there in the summer of 1969 which remains vivid in my mind as an example of the frenetic, bizarre nature of the times. The Center occupied the second and third floors of an old brownstone on the Near North Side of Chicago in a neighborhood then teeming with movement organizations. Two Weathermen collectives were housed close by, a "People's Park" grew out of the mud in a vacant lot across the street, and the Young Lord party had occupied a vacant church around the corner where they ran a day care center and an ongoing workshop in community organizing. The SHO members—two medical students taking time off and two women just out of nursing school—who staffed the Service Center suffered a continual and agonizing schizophrenia. Compared to the other neighborhood groups, they were comparatively rich with the tidy foundation grant. Their job was drab by any standards—the accumulation and redistribution of medical and political literature of possible interest to SHO chapters. Their mandate stopped there. The Weathermen and the Lords visited regularly, steadily increasing their demands for financial support. "The revolution is happening," their argument went, "and you're going to sit here packaging mailers pretending you're with us. Bullshit! Give us money." In 1969 in Chicago it was a tough line to rebut.

The day I visited we met to make some decisions about the future of the Center. It was hot Saturday in June and for reasons apparent only to Richard J. Daley, the Police Department had arbitrarily canceled a permit for a street dance that the Lords had planned for the evening in front of their church. As we met to discuss our mail order library, word spread of the cancellation and angry crowds began to assemble at the church. The police responded with D-Day psychology. Anything that could carry a cop was rolled into the streets surrounding the church. Motorcycles, paddy wagons, police cars, buses, and riot trucks occupied every inch of free curb space for blocks around. Hundreds of police in riot helmets lined the streets. Resolutely we attempted to discuss our problems while the din from the street grew. The Service Center staff, happy to vent their frustrations on someone, eagerly argued the "revolutionary" side of their schizophrenia. Why shouldn't they give the Service Center budget to the Weathermen or the Lords, they queried us? After all, the revolution *was* happening. With that the Chicago police moved in their final reinforcement—a helicopter. All afternoon the chopper wheeled to and fro in the sky over our meeting making discussion almost impossible. For a crazy moment it felt as if *the* revolution, *a* revolution, *some* revolution *was* happening.

Eventually the crowd, the cops, and the whirlybird all left without bloodshed or street dance. The Service Center limped along for another six or eight months before the coup de grace was delivered by a psychotic ex-Lord who stormed the office one day demanding money and, receiving none, filled the ceiling with lead. Nobody came back to work much after that. Like the SHO itself, the Service Center never really overcame its liberal university background. No longer satisfied with facile platitudes about the way life or medicine ought to be, but neither radicalized like the Weathermen nor a street organization like the Lords, the Service Center, like the SHO itself, withered and died, a victim of rapidly changing times.

During its mercurial five-year history the SHO did achieve a number of lasting changes. It made a strong case for relevance in health science education, lobbying for and accomplishing a host of curricular reforms. Most SHO-motivated reforms took place in medical schools where the focus and impact of the SHO was strongest, but parallel developments also occurred in nursing and dental education. The most striking success was the legitimatization of community medicine as a discipline. Many schools renovated antiquated Departments of Public Health or founded altogether new Departments of Community or Social Medicine under the direct influence of their students who had already been busy in the community. Other pressures (governmental expectations and survival politics among them) argued for increased medical school attention to the community and the society, but the interest, the experiences, and the demands of the SHO students of the mid-sixties has put social and community medicine in the curriculum of the seventies in a substantial and important way.

Beyond that the SHO succeeded in making student politics real. The SHO invited students to be not mere passive participants in their education and it demanded of the schools that the students be allowed to join in the community of scholars, the democratic university, which didn't mean dance committees and microscope exchanges. The SHO wanted in on the gut issues of the university—policy planning, student selection, and curriculum. Many schools relaxed their anti-student prejudices and included student representation on key committees. Certainly, students were listened to more carefully—if warily—during this period because their voices and sometimes their actions were strident.

When the SHO began to wane as an entity, of course, it relinquished its role as leader of the movement for student power on the health science campuses. Ironically and importantly, the custodian of dance committees and microscope exchanges, SAMA, was waiting to inherit the mantle of student relevance. SAMA had been energized by the rise of the SHO and the clear demonstration that there was an active political role for medical students in the medical school. SAMA survived the turbulence of the sixties and emerged with an activist leadership and some of the better principles and programs of the SHO. The rise and fall of the SHO left SAMA drastically changed and the heir to many of the solider reforms the SHO had achieved.

The SHO was a seminal experience for all of us involved in it. It stands as a counter medical education that remains more important for those of us who had it than the varieties of the traditional product that we experienced at our various schools. Under its influence medical school was a time of political growth and not just scientific training. As SHO graduates we became doctors committed to social and political change.

4

Slave to the Page Operator

The phone rang once and I was awake. "Yes," I said in a voice that invited more confidence than my soporific head deserved. "Dr. Mullan. This is the Delivery Room calling. Dr. Zigmund is about to deliver a woman who is extremely jaundiced. She has had no prenatal care and he doesn't know anything about her. He is worried about the condition of the fetus. Can you come quickly?" I struggled to get my mushy mind to focus on what she had told me. Delivery, jaundice, baby, help. The only thing I knew clearly was that I had to get out of bed. "Yes," I said again. "You do understand, Dr. Mullan, and you will come?" "Yes, yes," I answered.

Wearily I got to my feet, still tasting a late hospital supper. I pulled on my crumpled white pants and a stale shirt and walked out into the sultry July pre-dawn. The hospital was across the street. I was doing what they had told me I would do. I was an intern answering an emergency call in the middle of the night, tired, confused, and ill prepared.

I arrived at the Delivery Room and put my head in the door to ask what was happening. The obstetrical resident, Dr. Zigmund I supposed, also in his first month, yelled at me, "Get changed and get your ass back in here. She's a multip, complete, and coming fast." I saw no more of the patient than her brown-yellow bottom on the delivery table. I obeyed.

When I arrived back in my baggy scrub suit the woman was ready to give birth and the air of near hysteria in the room had peaked. As I fumblingly opened and set up my pediatric emergency kit, I looked at the woman. She was a handsome, tan, Puerto Rican who looked older than her twenty-five years. There was an unmistakable jaundice to her skin and the whites of her eyes glowed yellow. She spoke no English. Stoically she bore the rending pains of the final minutes of childbirth, allowing only an occasional "aye-yay-yay-yay" to escape her lips. "I think it's hepatitis," Zigmund told me. "She just walked in off the street. No prenatal care. Nothing. The fetal heart is okay but when she's this jaundiced who knows what the baby will be like."

I certainly didn't. I knew little about hepatitis in the adult and nothing about the disease in the newborn. I couldn't call the resident who was still asleep. There was no time. The baby was on its way. I had seen an infant resuscitated once in the Delivery Room but I had never tried it myself. I arranged my tubes, my blades, and my collection of chemicals. Then I waited.

Zigmund delivered the infant quickly and with skill. It started to squall while still in the birth canal and howled mightily by the time Zigmund held him aloft, a frothy brown trophy. Fortunately, no fancy pediatrics and no resuscitation were needed. The child did not appear jaundiced and a call to the resident, who came wearily over to examine our new charge, confirmed that hepatitis in the mother is rarely a problem for the newborn.

Fearfully, proudly, idealistically, I became an intern. Happy to be finally pursuing the profession I had agonized over for so long, naggingly aware that many critics of medicine pointed to internship as the point in the physician's career when principle turns to avarice, when self-sacrifice becomes self-service, I went to work.

I chose pediatrics as my specialty because children seemed to me infinitely more salvageable than adults and therefore worthy of more pains and more interest. Sparing an infant the discomfort and damage of a disease appealed to me because the return would be enjoyed for a lifetime, perhaps sixty or seventy years, as opposed to the benefit that would fall briefly to an adult—maybe twenty, maybe five, maybe one year. Then and since I have been asked frequently, "But isn't it horrible when a child dies?" Of course the answer is yes, but luckily it happens only rarely and is more than offset by the spectacular powers of resilience children possess. Children would be fun, I speculated, and they were.

For internship I chose Jacobi Hospital, a municipal institution in the Northeast Bronx affiliated with Albert Einstein College of Medicine. I went to Jacobi because it was in New York, my home, because it enjoyed a good academic reputation and, most of all, because it was a public hospital. Unlike most cities where a single, mammoth municipal hospital predominates (the names call forth both awe and horror: Cook County, San Francisco General, Boston City, D.C.

General, etc.), New York supports a "system" of municipal hospitals. They range from the famous (Bellevue) to the notorious (Harlem), from the respected (Kings County) to the unknown (Greenpoint). At a distance, in medical school, two things occurred to me. First, it seemed that New York took a much more progressive approach to the medical problems of its citizens than did most American cities. Given a hospital system second only to the military in size and budget, this seemed a plausible conclusion. Where else could one go in the United States and be part of a medical system that was attempting to deal in some coherent way with the health problems of the poor and indigent? Second, I was long overdue for working in a public hospital. As ardent a critic as I had become of the medical care rendered the poor, I had never worked in an institution whose primary goal was the provision of that care. Alone among Chicago's medical schools, the University of Chicago had no affiliation with Cook County Hospital. All of my medical training had taken place on the very private floors of the university medical center, Billings Hospital.

Jacobi Hospital rises a stolid ten floors out of a meadow in the far reaches of the Bronx. Using subways, buses, and beat-up cars from ghettos closer to the heart of the city, many blacks and Puerto Ricans find themselves in the wooded suburban affluence of Pelham Parkway heading toward "their" hospital. The community surrounding Jacobi is white, Jewish or Italian, middle class. They have little use for the hospital and resent the steady passage of people of color through their neighborhood. They call on the hospital only for their emergencies and, sometimes, for their elderly. The average member of the community proudly relies for his care on a patchwork of private doctors and small private hospitals. Receiving hospital, medical center, teaching facility, Jacobi is in no way a community hospital for any identifiable neighborhood—least of all its own.

As interns we spent one hundred hours a week in the hospital. We worked a six-day week and were on call in the hospital every other night; we had ample time to become familiar with the hospital. Jacobi had a certain smell to it. Built in the days before central air-conditioning, it seemed the same well-used air ebbed and flowed down the long inner hallways of the large building for months at a time. Now aseptic, now ever so slightly putrid, the Jacobi odor was richest and stalest in the basement where smells from poorly washed garbage cans and from the employees' cafeteria flowed together. In summer the heat became so intense at the center of the building that waiting for an elevator became a sweaty chore. One staff member, in an act notable both for its rank individualism as well as for its reasonableness, walled off the cubicle assigned him as an office and installed an air-conditioner with its exhaust aimed into the corridor. During the long summer months we were insulted by his hot air pouring out into the already steamy hallway.

My recollections of Jacobi are dominated by the sensation of my baggy white uniform. On the first day of internship every new arrival received six square-cut, styleless white pants designed to fit three or four sizes, with jackets to match. The uniforms were part of our six-line contract that assured us a wage ($4,500 then), meals, and laundry services in return for our travail. The laundry proved short on soap but well stocked with starch, the uniforms often being returned with the bloodstains ironed in and the pants starched so they would barely bend. Treading the halls of the hospital in my stovepipe pants, I remember mostly tired feet and bulging pockets—the intern's saddle bags. They transported reprints of journal articles, a stethoscope, a pen flashlight, a stack of file cards bearing patients' names and chores to be done, pens, tourniquets, alcohol swabs, and tongue depressors. I was always tired. A vague nausea and a cotton dryness in my mouth were the taste of a night without sleep—a frequent experience. It is hard to measure the exact toll that exhaustion claimed on my mental processes. I always seemed to respond in some manner in a medical crisis. But as I became more tired the flavor in my mouth gradually changed, serving as an indicator, most likely, of mental deterioration as well.

Meaningless tragedy dogged the intern's steps as much as high drama and all-night heroics. For several months I cared for a child we called "Hot Dog." Hot Dog had been a normal four-year-old boy who choked while eating a hot dog many months before. The meat lodged in his windpipe and by the time it had been cleared he suffered severe and permanent brain damage. Now he lived in the pediatric ward, gnarled beyond recognition, fed by a stomach tube, the subject of occasional, pitiful, speechless visits from his parents. We had to call him "Hot Dog." We who had to deal with him everyday could not afford the tears or the depression of his parents. He was too real to us and we had to use humor, a hardened, grim wit, for our own defense. Mercifully, senselessly, he died one night. I felt relief.

Death in children was not always so easy to take. Maria Rodriguez also lived in the pediatric ward. Stunted by the ravages of a relentless kidney disease, she looked two or three years younger than her actual age of eleven. She boarded with us because her kidneys had shut down altogether and without the benefit of a twice weekly visit to a dialysis machine she would have died quickly. Her arm always wrapped in a large bandage that protected the artery and vein exposed for the convenience of the machine, she roamed and danced the hospital corridors, a beautiful, mischievous, pert child. She answered the phone at the Nursing Station ("Eight West, Miss Rodriquez speaking"), followed us on rounds, stealing stethoscopes and tying interns' shoelaces to bedposts, and welcomed new children to the floor like a member of the Lilliput chamber of commerce. She died and it was crushing. Two efforts at kidney transplant failed and she succumbed to complications the second time. None of us talked about her for many months.

Death haunted us even when it didn't happen. I spent an intense forty-eight-hour period working with a six-year-old mauled in an auto accident. Although his condition remained critical for much of the time, it became clear at the end of the second day that he would live. The parents, who had hovered outside the room for the entire ordeal, were overjoyed. Leaving the child's care to another intern, I said goodnight to the family and started for the elevator to go home. The boy's father, a small Puerto Rican man who spoke little English, stopped me and without ceremony pressed a ten-dollar bill into my hand. I protested vehemently and tried to give the money back. The city paid me a good salary, I argued, and while I appreciated his generosity I could not in conscience accept his money. I knew all the while that ten dollars was a substantial gift on his part and one that he could ill afford. He firmly refused to take the money back and after several efforts it became apparent that my attempts to return the crumpled bill were insulting to him. At length I kept the tip, feeling the damage would be worse if I persevered in my effort to return it. Riding down in the elevator, feeling both flattered and embarrassed, it suddenly occurred to me that the child still might die. Then how would the ten dollars feel in my pocket and how would I be able to live with the family or myself? I took the next elevator up and bluntly shoved the bill back into the father's hand, stating that keeping the money could jeopardize my job. I won that round but when the boy left the hospital several weeks later the family presented me with a beautiful briefcase with "DR. MULLAN" embossed on the side. I still use it proudly and I am sure it cost a good deal more than ten dollars.

As an experience, internship has certain strengths. It goes without saying that it is a period of intensity—intense learning, intense exposure to patients and disease, and intense testing of one's own strength and stamina. In many ways the intensity is good. At the least, it is an experience matched by few life situations—the line of battle, the religious retreat, childbirth, perhaps acute temporary illness or insanity. But few life circumstances parallel internship for duration of demand on the individual.

I cannot deny that the intimacy achieved during internship with people and with disease processes is a unique and a valuable experience. Living and working for forty-eight hours with a person crippled by asthma teaches more about the disease than any text ever could. Laboring over a child suffering severe croup and dealing with the family while the illness becomes steadily worse and then, miraculously, abates tells more about the human condition than the best of novels. There is no simple substitute that I can think of for this kind of education, and it is an education that is at least relevant and, probably, essential to being a physician.

Moreover, the physical challenge of internship teaches a brand of confidence that is helpful under stress. Finishing internship, I knew that I was prepared to work at all hours of the day or night, I had learned what it was to be called out of bed and into action at three in the morning, and the dawn had been demystified for me. For better or for worse, I knew I could work steadily for twenty-four or thirty-six hours if necessary.

My life came to revolve around internship. A few short years before, I had objected to my afternoons being consumed by science labs. Now medical chores occupied my days and nights, my week and weekends. Like all my fellow interns, my free time was oriented primarily to catching up on sleep. We grumbled but we accepted this situation with little or no challenge. Somehow we were there, the children were sick, others were doing it, others had done it, and we accepted.

This acquiescence is very much part of becoming a doctor. The absolute destruction of the nine-to-five mentality enables the practicing physician to labor at whatever hour of the day or night he is called. Without this flexibility, without this casualness about time, patients would go untended or doctors would go crazy. If I had suffered the same anguish that I experienced going to organic chemistry lab every time I was called in the middle of the night as an intern, I would have folded in the first month. In traditional terms, internship bred devotion to patients and dedication to job. But really, it was more than this. Commitment became a state of mind, a reflex. We were totally involved with people and their many illnesses.

Yet this same acquiescence cost all of us personally. Two days after I graduated from medical school and three weeks before starting internship I got married. Judy and I came to New York excited about our new life together. We rented an apartment in the far reaches of the Bronx not because it was an area in which either of us wanted to live but because it was close to the hospital. We decorated it and moved in our few pieces of furniture, which did not include a bed that was still on order. When it came it was too wide for the steps that led to our basement dwelling—a crushing event for both of us—and we had to sleep on the floor for several more weeks. After ten days of nest building I left for the hospital. Every second night I would come home weary and often preoccupied. Every other weekend I worked all weekend, which meant Judy and I parted at 7:30 Saturday morning and I came home again at about 6:00 on Monday night, a schedule hardly good for friendship, let alone intimacy. Every time I was on duty at the hospital I faithfully stole ten late-night minutes to call home and report the events of the day. That was our only contact for thirty-six hours—thirty-six hours that happened three times a week.

Judy had a degree in biochemistry and had worked at the University of Chicago doing lipid research. She was dissatisfied with lab science, though, and moving to New York she hoped to find a job working with people rather than test tubes. For six months she looked for employment in the general area of social welfare but without a degree or any experience in the field, work was hard to find. Finally she took the only job she could come by—a job she thought she would dislike and she did. She became a welfare worker for the City of New York.

The general situation was disappointing to me too. The close friendship Judy and I had had for a year was diluted by internship. It was as if I had undergone two marriages at once—to a woman by choice and to a hospital by contract and custom. During that first year I had less time than Judy to think about what was happening, but we are both clear now that internship was a greedy mistress and placed a heavy toll on our marriage. Judy remains articulate on the subject. Unemployed much of the year, alone much of the time in a community far from any she would have chosen to live in, virtually widowed shortly after her wedding, occasional housekeeper for a zombie, she feels that year was one of the worst of her life. Our marriage, coming as it did at the very outset of internship, made the problem more dramatic than it might have been, but internship, I am convinced, is a severe trial for any couple.

That first year of medicine also borrowed a bit of my humanity— a debt I doubt will ever be repaid. The job required the mechanization and routinization of my life. Every aspect of my existence, from when I made rounds to draw blood in the early morning to when I stole five minutes to go to the bathroom, had to be carefully planned. The absolute volume of chores as well as the human responsibilities of an intern dictate that life be parsimoniously meted out so that the multiple jobs get done. I had to give up many pastimes that I had enjoyed in previous years. I rarely had time or energy for any sports. Judy bought us opera tickets for our anniversary and I slept through *La Bohème*—in a $17 seat. I was bathed daily in the drama of human life but rarely recorded any of what I saw, though I had enjoyed writing in earlier years. I thought about these things as they were happening to me and consoled myself that internship was a temporary state of affairs and that my momentarily caged spirit would rebound when the year was over. Of course internship was followed by residency which, while not quite so oppressive, featured the same sort of demands and constraints. The discipline that house officership (internship and residency together) teaches is, as I have suggested, important to the practice of clinical medicine. But the intensity of experience to which I was subjected, the degree to which my life was bludgeoned and bent by the demands of the hospital has done more to me than simply teach medical discipline. The spirit cannot escape unaltered from such an ordeal. Like a factory worker who can no longer hear high notes because he has been partially deafened by the roar of machinery, I worry about my own sensitivity to people and to life. Internship remains with me today, I am sure, as more than just a memory.

I often asked myself why internship existed. Surely, I said in discouraged or exhausted moments, there must be a better way of doing business than this. In truth, there is no better way of doing *business* than the present structure of internship. There are, as I have outlined, various academic arguments for the one-hundred-hour week for interns. Some, in my judgment, have merit. The financial arguments for the present way of doing things are rarely articulated, exceedingly clear (far clearer than the academic reasons), and extremely sinister. The terms of internship, of course, vary somewhat from place to place and, to be sure, have been improving in recent years, but the facts I will outline pertain by and large. The same circumstances apply to residency as well.

House officers,* once reimbursed with laundry and free meals, are now paid a respectable $10,000 per year on the average. Clearly the experience has educational aspects that enable the young physician to garner skills for which he or she will be paid well in later life. But any hospital administrator knows that the intern or resident is no average employee. When everybody else is punching out to go home, the interns and residents on duty are settling in to cover the night. The administrator knows he has a stable of double- to triple-duty workers that he can count on. Moreover, these are no ordinary workers. They have credentials (if not always skills) that enable them to do the work of nurses, orderlies, and lab techs. The slack, the administrator knows, will always be picked up by the interns and residents who, if necessary, can start I.V.'s, give shots, pass pills, turn patients, draw blood, analyze urines, push patients to X-ray, ride the ambulance, and so on. The $10,000 per year for an intern or resident is money exceedingly well spent by the hospital.

House officers work from 80 to 120 hours a week with no overtime pay and no compensatory days off. If an intern stays up all night with a patient he doesn't take the next morning off for sleep. He simply continues working until it is time to go home. He is an employer's dream. The house officer spends twice as much time in the hospital as any other employee, making him, on an hourly basis, the poorest paid worker in the medical center. Given his range of skills, he is a fabulous buy.

The message of this analysis is not that interns and residents should be paid double or triple what they are now. Their wages are, I think, quite reasonable. Rather the significance of these facts lies in their import for the rest of the hospital and for patient care. While most administrators are not so malevolent as to consciously exploit the house staff, many fall comfortably into it. Economy clearly invites the reduction of "ancillary" staff and, where house staff will be on duty all the time, the temptation to skimp on other staffing is omnipresent. This situation is at its worst in city hospitals where budget problems are chronic and the house staff is often large. It certainly stands out as a major factor in my experience at two city hospitals, Jacobi and Lincoln.

* The terms house officer and house staff, which will be used interchangeably, refer to interns and residents as a group.

Hospital floors of thirty and forty patients were frequently covered by a single nurse for eight-hour shifts, meaning that we stayed with any patients who were really ill. After five o'clock we rarely had messenger service in the hospital and, as a result, we pushed our patients to X-ray, carried specimens to the lab, brought our new patients from the Emergency Room, and so on. The impact of this situation on patient care was obvious; it was slower and sloppier than it need have been. Clearer yet was the implication of this state of affairs for other workers in the hospital. Messengers could be laid off, nurses turned away, orderlies furloughed, and lab techs dropped since the hospital had an ever-present complement of interns and residents who, if pressed, would do the jobs of many of the other workers. Hospitals can run cheaply, if not smoothly, with house staff plugging the holes.

The implications of this system were not lost on us and we felt exploited by it. Often, so often, we felt abandoned by the system and yet responsible for it. The administrators had gone home, nurses were missing, the Intensive Care Unit was full, machinery wasn't working, lab tests were unavailable, and we had to practice medicine; we had to answer to patients and their families. We monitored the acutely ill in the absence of nurses by staying up all night at the bedside. We wrote our examinations and consultations out in longhand because dictating equipment was not available. We analyzed bloods and urines ourselves because the one technician in the lab was overwhelmed. We could—and did—support the system with our own work, our own sleep, and our own lives.

As a group, young physicians emerge from the intern resident experience changed by it. To a very considerable extent, house officership contributes to greed among physicians. The years after medical school, marked as they are by long hours, tough working conditions and, particularly in the past, poor pay, stimulate the most avaricious side of the medical graduate. Many physicians spend their careers extracting reparations from a society that has forced them through a painful rite of passage. I cannot deny that I bear grudges for the quantities of my life given over to the hospital during my training. The humanization of house officership (including better working conditions, fewer hours on duty, and reasonable pay) would help to change the personality of the medical profession in future years. Doctors less browbeaten in their formative years would be more likely and more able to keep their minds set on the principled goals that often brought them into medicine in the first place. At the least, they would leave training and enter practice looking and behaving less like the Veterans of Foreign Wars.

Many of my fellow interns at Jacobi agreed that the system of medicine that we were living and supporting was abusive in many ways. We focused not so much on our own problems (as I have suggested, we generally accepted the intern's way of life) as we did on what the system did to people using it—the patients. My own honeymoon with municipal medicine, the happy system of socialized health care I expected to find when I came to New York, was short-lived. Care at Jacobi was woefully impersonal. The hospital was governed by the adjacent medical school, Albert Einstein, which meant that the priorities in the city facility were those of teaching and research rather than community service. No community input or control existed in any form. Understaffing and resultant abuses of patient care flourished everywhere. As interns we had little to say about these circumstances even though many of them affected us directly. About the middle of the year, however, an edict came along that rankled us and that we thought deserved some resistance. A typed memo arrived from the administrators' office stating that a visit to the Emergency Room would now cost sixteen dollars instead of ten dollars. No reference was made as to why. There was no sliding scale, no prior notification, no community approval. Of course these were not considerations to which the hospital ever paid attention. But we thought they should and so we decided to fight the fee increase.

Among the eighteen pediatric interns at Jacobi there were a number who had been student activists. Steve Sharfstein and Herb Schreier, both Einstein graduates and both destined to become psychiatrists, served with me as co-captains of the fee battle. Marty Stein, from Los Angeles, who had been a close friend since the first SHO convention in Chicago, was an intern classmate and a strong supporter of the fight. Barbara Blase, from Buffalo, was in our ranks as was Julie Ingelfinger, an old college friend, Einstein graduate, and SHO activist. The entire group of pediatric interns was supportive of the action and, after a council of war during which the director of the department agreed to look the other way, we began a noisy campaign telling our patients not to pay their bills. We posted signs in the waiting area, handed leaflets to patients, and urged everybody not to pay when they left. Sharfstein, Schreier, and I, wearing our baggy intern outfits, went on camera. We called a press conference in the Pediatric Emergency Room and, much to our astonishment, two television networks, a host of radio stations, and New York's three daily papers showed up and squeezed in to cover the story.

It made great copy: "Doctors Tell Patients Not to Pay Bills." Who had ever heard of such a thing? New York was interested and the hospital administration was staggered. They had given little thought to their new fees and certainly had never experienced or expected a mutiny from their medical staff on a subject like patient-billing. In all likelihood the policy governing the new rates originated downtown at the Department of Hospitals and they simply published it as directed. Suddenly the hospital was in the glare of TV lights. Who determined fees, the press wanted to know? How did they justify sixteen dollars per visit? Why was patient income not taken into account when charges were set? The confrontation, it became clear, cost them more in exposure and embarrassment than the increased charges would ever net. On the third day they backed down, reinstating the old fee and promising a sliding scale based on income if charges were increased in the future. We were jubilant.

Our next scrape was a tougher one. During the fee battle most of the staff of the hospital stood back and watched with interested skepticism. The formal House Staff Association for instance, declined to support the campaign because, they said, it had not gone through proper channels. Our victory, though, converted many of the observers as became clear later that spring when the Department of Hospitals announced budget cuts that would curtail a number of services at Jacobi. Budget cuts in a large institution are usually handled quietly and craftily by the city. The primary weapon is what is called a "job freeze." This means that when a worker resigns or retires no one is hired to fill the slot. The result is a smaller payroll for the city (without firing anyone), more work for the remaining staff, and poorer service for the patient. A job freeze was on the agenda for Jacobi. Moreover a number of services would be curtailed or shut down. The hospital, for instance, had a special Intensive Care Unit for burn victims. It was to be closed. Certain lab tests were to be dropped and others were to be rationed on a Monday, Wednesday, Friday schedule. And so forth. The House Staff Association (the organization representative of all the interns and residents in the hospital), asking the pediatric interns for guidance, immediately voted to oppose the cuts. Moreover, the Medical Board (the organization of senior physicians at the hospital) announced similar sentiments and let it be known that they would willingly join in some form of job action to dramatize the cuts. Finally, and perhaps most important, we were approached by the leaders of the Drug and Hospital Workers, Local 1199, the union representing a significant percentage of the hospital workers at Jacobi. Their sentiments also ran toward concerted job action.

We were an unlikely and probably unprecedented troika. Abe Dimmer, the 1199 leader, was the primary philosopher and strategist of the movement. Longshoreman turned lab tech, long-time political activist, veteran of street brawls and picket lines, he led our planning sessions with sensitivity and clarity. "We are fighting for medical care," he would say, "and we are fighting for our jobs. We must win. We have no choice." Dr. Joe Forzano, surgeon, professor, registered Republican, denizen of Westchester County, spoke for the Medical Board. Generally he was more militant than Dimmer. "We've taken enough crap. We've got to make a stand for city hospitals or get out of them."

Job actions in hospitals are tricky affairs. Traditional industrial strikes aim to punish the employer far more than the consumer. But hospital strikes that curtail services run the risk of damaging the consumer—the patient—directly, an embarrassment the management can bear and, often, turn back against the strikers. Since our protest concerned the curtailment of patient care we obviously did not want to hurt the patient in the process. Nonetheless, the budget cuts would diminish patient care considerably. The city banked on the fact that, as in all human services, attrition and piecemeal cuts in program would pass unnoticed by an unorganized public. Our strategy, under Dimmer's guidance, became the exposure of the cuts and what they would mean over the months to come. We agreed upon a dramatic scheme that would, in truth, produce more smoke than fire. Two weeks in advance, we announced the closure of the hospital. We held a press conference that, again, received good coverage, distributed pamphlets, and contacted local politicians to enlist support. On the announced morning the main floor of the hospital was turned into a giant Emergency Room with an elaborate triage system functioning to separate people who were really ill from those with a minor complaint or a routine visit scheduled. Physicians from every department participated, evaluating all arrivals with a speed and efficiency rarely seen in the hospital on normal workdays. Attending physicians worked alongside interns and residents screening new patients. The entire hospital staff—medical and nonmedical—in fact worked together with esprit and animation. Shop stewards from 1199 and professors from the medical school, residents from surgery, and technicians from the labs worked side by side to coordinate the action. Anyone with pain or with signs of significant illness was transferred to a second area where they were examined and treated appropriately. Patients were admitted when necessary and the hospital floors functioned in a routine manner. Anybody with a minor complaint or anyone coming for a routine outpatient visit was given a handful of literature explaining the situation and sent home. Response was mixed. Irate, some people took the time to dress us down before swearing they would never return to Jacobi no matter what the budget. Others understood the situation and carried leaflets home with them or joined with us in talking to new arrivals. The press generally covered the story sympathetically.

We again succeeded in embarrassing the city. Hospital budgets had always been determined centrally and aside from an occasional protest by a beleaguered administrator or department chairman, nobody ever challenged the authority of the city over the management of "their" hospitals. Certainly the entire clientele of a hospital had never been exhorted to write the mayor and call the City Council to demand better funding for a municipal institution. And the stakes were high, much higher than the sixteen-dollar fee issue. If the workers ("professional" and "nonprofessional") as well as the patients from a hospital could join together to demand better funding, what aspect of city management would remain inviolable? It was a populist revolt, with the workers and patients demanding to set the hospital priorities rather than the politicians and the budget makers. More than the money concerned, the action itself was a threat to the city administration. The city had a principle to defend—their right to determine the fate and style of city medicine free of the encumbrances of worker, patient, and community opinion.

The city moved quickly and cleverly. New York's mayor, John Lindsay, much quoted on the subject of neighborhood government and citizen input, officially ignored the issue. Worried, in fact, about an upcoming bid for re-election, he wanted no disruption in the area of health and hospitals and, doubtless, gave the green light to his administrators to do what they could to quash the insurrection. The Department of Hospitals reckoned accurately that the Achilles heel of the job action was neither the notoriously independent union nor the angry house staff. Rather they singled out the senior staff, the Medical Board. The city's approach was indirect and cunning. The city knew that all the members of the Medical Board who ran the various departments at Jacobi were also faculty members of Albert

Einstein College of Medicine and generally deeply committed to the medical school. Over the years the city had given the medical school large grants annually to "staff" Jacobi—that is, to pay Albert Einstein faculty members to work at Jacobi. This was the mechanism for tying the medical school into the city hospital. These grants were large and generally poorly monitored by the city. There had always been rumors around Jacobi and Einstein about certain professors and researchers paid with city money who weren't seen at Jacobi from one year to the next. The city apparently had been checking on the use of its money. Neither 1199 nor the house staff group was approached by the Commissioner of Hospitals. Rather, it seemed that the city's "message" was delivered through the dean of the medical school, Harry Gordon. Gordon, a noted pediatric researcher and the custodian of the interests of the medical school, was not prepared for a showdown with the city. He understood the message and responded predictably.

Three days into the hospital "closure" I represented the house staff at an emergency meeting of the Medical Board called by Dr. Gordon, not at Jacobi, but in his office at the medical school. "End the strike," he urged flatly. "It is damaging the medical school and things could get a lot worse." Those members of the Medical Board who were ambivalent about the job action to begin with rushed to back the dean. But the Board as a whole followed the firm line enunciated by Dr. Forzano and took no action to reverse the closure. Over the next two days rumors began to circulate about what the city had on the medical school and what would happen if they released it. At the end of that time a second Medical Board meeting was held from which house staff and union members were excluded. The dean apparently outlined the potential damage to the medical school in vivid terms and effectively broke the back of any principled resistance. The Medical Board voted unilaterally to reopen the hospital the following Monday, three days distant. At nine o'clock that Monday morning the house staff met and argued the question for almost an hour. Two hundred interns and residents (two-thirds of the house staff) showed up for the heated debate. The first vote taken was narrowly in favor of continuing the closure without the support of the Medical Board. But since everyone knew chaos would reign in a hospital with a divided house staff, a second vote produced a majority in favor of capitulation. The union, feeling it could not go it alone, followed the lead of the house staff and returned to work. We were beaten.

So the budget cuts came. Clerks were laid off, the lab stopped doing certain blood tests and rationed others, the burn unit closed, and so on. The average patient arriving at the sprawling hospital complex never knew the difference. Before long there were new interns and much of the staff had moved on. The budget fight of 1969 was largely forgotten. But there were lessons to be drawn from it. The most immediate conclusions were made by the lab techs, clerks, and orderlies who were laid off as well as by those who stayed behind, since their jobs were made more demanding by the departure of their fellows. For them the lesson—not really a new one—was that the system was capricious and all they could carry home was a bitterness.

Local 1199 concluded that doctors were not to be relied upon politically. The union had always considered the city and the medical school their adversaries. Doctors as a group had never particularly figured in their concept of the battle for income and job security. "We had no position on docs," Dimmer mused. "But this was an unusual bunch of them. We thought it would be worth a try. Sort of a *united front*. We got burned. Now we know what we knew to begin with: our strength is ourselves, our rank and file. It won't happen again."

I did not agree entirely with the veteran labor leader. To be sure, the Medical Board had been the weak link in our "united front." It was disappointing that we had not been able to hold on longer but, nonetheless, doctors striking for hospital services was something new. The younger physicians—the house staff—had remained militant in defense of the action until the end. This was something different from the individualism, the privatism, the self-seeking that has so often characterized doctors' political efforts. The Jacobi house staff had been willing to undertake highly visible, controversial action at potential hazard to themselves. Perhaps from a labor standpoint the doctors weren't tough, but the doctors were doing something doctors hadn't done before and that was significant.

On the other hand it was true that the physicians (senior and junior) who worked at Jacobi did not have the same stake in the hospital that many of the hospital workers did. The house staff was transient, spending from one to four years at the institution for training. The senior physicians had their identities divided between the city hospital and the medical school with, as they demonstrated, final allegiance going to the school. Most significant, perhaps, was the fact that none of the physicians used Jacobi as their hospital. When a surgeon needed surgery, when an intern's wife was to deliver, when a resident contracted hepatitis, they invariably used the College Hospital or some other private facility in the city. None of the medical staff and none of their families were ever at risk at Jacobi as patients. Jacobi was their work place but when they got sick they went elsewhere.

The members of 1199 and the other hospital workers differed from the physicians in their relation to the hospital in two significant ways. First, Jacobi was their job and their only job. Many had been there for years and intended to remain. Jacobi was their employment security. They had no divided allegiances. Second, most of the hospital workers used Jacobi for their medical care and that of their families. They knew the hospital, they knew the doctors, and the services were available to them. All told, their stake in Jacobi was considerably greater than that of the doctors.

Dimmer was right: the doctors were different from the workers he represented. But what did this mean for future confrontations? What did this mean for doctors as a labor force or a source of reform within the medical system? Did their special position within the system invalidate them as real workers or as agents of progressive change? These questions troubled me particularly because they began to eat away at some pat and romantic notions I had carried with me from the days of the SHO. In medical school the press had called us the "New Breed." I had assumed, as many of us had, that we really were representatives of a new generation of physicians different in kind from our predecessors. More liberal than previous generations of young doctors, exposed in growing numbers to campus protest and unrest, soon to be better paid than house officers ever had been, the interns and residents of 1970 were not carbon copies of previous generations. Yet the belief in a new breed of doctor was overly dramatic. Confrontation was the style of the time and with appropriate leadership house staff could be induced to take stands that appeared militant, populist, radical. But that did not make interns and residents the agents of revolution. House staff would argue with the system but they were not ready to overthrow it.

In the late 1950s several interns and residents from New York's municipal hospital system came together and hired a lawyer to represent them in a variety of grievances they had with the city. By the late 1960s this group had grown into the Committee of Interns and Residents (CIR), a loosely organized citywide union of house staff that carried on contract negotiations with the city and generally tried to look after house staff interests. I had attempted in vain to enlist their support in the sixteen-dollar fee issue and, in the process, had become involved in their politics. By the time of the budget-cut action I had been voted the Jacobi representative to the citywide body.

By labor standards, the CIR was a primitive union in 1969. Other than a dollar per pay period dues that primarily covered the retainer fee of our lawyer, the group had little organization. Every hospital had its own system of producing a delegate who frequently, though not always, attended a monthly meeting at the lawyer's office for the purpose of conducting business. Business usually consisted of the ongoing details of the intern-resident contract with the city. At that point the CIR had no publications nor any educational or social function. There was as yet no self-consciousness on the part of house officers that would suggest to their organization any of these activities. The handful of delegates to the CIR (the only house officers from different hospitals in the city to meet regularly with each other) never got together without their lawyer and, actually, never convened outside of his Lower Broadway office.

To his great credit, Murray Gordon, the CIR's attorney, had the prescience to see physicians—house staff in particular—as an organized labor force when no one else dreamed of it. Gordon was involved with the CIR from the start and as generation of house officer succeeded generation, he became the constant force in the organization. Veteran labor lawyer, seasoned in New York politics, respected adversary and friend of the city's labor negotiators, Gordon generally towered above any group of interns and residents in aplomb and savvy. Over the years he had developed a fairly fixed notion of what house staff politics should be. Interns and residents were an exploited class of workers. Collective bargaining (unionization) had been the way out for other city hospital workers and the house staff should follow suit. He organized the CIR and governed its business down through the years with that goal in mind. Every two years or so the intern and resident contract came up for renegotiation and the CIR under Gordon's tutelage pushed house staff wages and benefits forward.

The name Murray Gordon would have meant nothing to the majority of interns and residents in New York throughout this period. The CIR itself would have been known only vaguely to them as being responsible for pay increases in some manner or other. Most signed a card at the beginning of the year at the urging of their hospital representative pledging a dollar a pay period and then forgot about it. They expected no newsletters, business meetings, symposia, or political positions—and they got none. They joined the CIR in the hope of higher salaries and they weren't often disappointed.

Actually, by the late sixties the salary negotiation had grown formal on both sides. The city had an Office of Collective Bargaining with whom we did business. First we would hold long debates among the CIR delegates about what income levels we should demand and eventually arrived at figures close to those suggested by Gordon in the first place. In turn, he would pass these on to the city. Much backroom discussion would then take place between our counselor and the city representatives and then he would return to us with their counterproposal, usually well short of our price. Somewhere along the line we would travel to an upper floor of an office building with a good view overlooking City Hall Park and the East River and lock horns rather ceremoniously with the city negotiators. We always came dressed in our baggy whites with stethoscopes hanging out of our pockets, stressing the vital nature of our work and suggesting that we might be called away at any moment (like firemen coming with their helmets and axes). We banged the table, looked angry (which some of us were), and dropped hints about job actions and not being able to control "the men." Then we retired and Gordon again disappeared with the city negotiators. Eventually, figures were agreed upon which we took back to the hospitals and, usually, sold to "the men" without much difficulty because they always represented substantial gains.

The trouble with the CIR up to that point was that it was a single-issue organization—bread and butter for the troops. It made no pretenses of being a "professional organization," it hardly communicated with its membership, and its politics were limited to protecting its monetary gains. House officers, though, were changing and it seemed to me reasonable—even likely—that their organization would change too. The house staff at Jacobi had been more activist and more dramatic in the course of a year than any group in the history of the CIR. Moreover, the CIR delegates generally sympathized with the Jacobi positions. Confrontation politics were popular in the late sixties and young physicians, no matter what their social attitudes, were not immune to the appeal of direct action. Murray Gordon was not at all enthusiastic about hospital confrontations, especially over issues that did not arise directly out of the CIR's contract, but the delegates were definitely interested. Although they balked at supporting the sixteen-dollar fee battle, the organization heartily endorsed the budget-cut fight and Jacobi's "closure." In word, at least, the CIR had backed direct-action politics in support of a non-salary issue.

After a year and a half as the Jacobi delegate I was elected president of the CIR. (Election, again, was by delegates and not by membership.) All the delegates knew where I stood on social action versus salaries. My reputation was worse than I deserved. I felt that if enough of them voted for me to elect me then there was a consensus to use the CIR as a vehicle for change in the city hospitals. A number of the delegates felt as strongly as I did about new directions for the CIR. The Bellevue representative, for instance, was an internal medicine resident who counted himself a devout Marxist. In the context of the CIR he limited his dialectics and his tendency toward soap boxing and worked hard and consistently for patient-care programs. The delegate from Coney Island always struck me as more of a taxicab driver than a doctor. He labored under a heavy New York accent, a penchant for banging his fist on the table at negotiations, and a tendency to talk out of the side of his mouth. Salaries had always been his primary concern but conditions at his hospital had gotten to him and he became an ardent publicist of hospital conditions.

As a group we worked out a two-pronged strategy to make the CIR a force in the debates surrounding patient care and hospital conditions. The first half of our strategy involved our contract with the city, an area that Murray Gordon disapproved of from the start. The CIR contract expired in the fall of 1970 and as part of the new contract we sought and received the approval of the delegate body for two new clauses. The first asked that the city guarantee that a given ratio of nurses and messengers to house officers be on duty in all hospitals at all times so that house officers would not have to do "out of title" work—a favorite and frequent complaint of other city unions. The second clause asked that a minimum set of laboratory tests be available on a twenty-four-hour basis in all the hospitals so that we could practice "standardized, up-to-date medicine." The city negotiators rejected these at our very first session saying that these were "management issues," not appropriate to the contract of employees. We, of course, had the choice of arguing these points further or dropping them. Our counselor argued strenuously that the city would not yield and that we were only jeopardizing potential contract benefits. Our moral arguments fared poorly against such pragmatism and the majority of delegates voted to drop the "patient-care demands" from the second round of negotiations. The first prong of our two-pronged program had failed.

The other half of the program lived longer. We conceived of what we came to call a Registry of Abuse—the compilation of a file of hospital misplays caused not by malice or intentional malpractice but by inadequate staffing, insufficient or obsolete equipment that resulted in undue suffering or death to patients. The delegates liked the idea and agreed that the CIR should collect the incident reports from its members and make the file known to the Department of Hospitals. If no remedial action was taken, they resolved, the CIR would make the horror stories public. I announced the initiation of the registry at a press conference at City Hall and received front-page coverage in the *New York Times*. The idea fascinated the press and worried many people in the municipal hierarchy. Unfortunately, the concept left house officers cold. After six months and many pleas for reports, we compiled four—two of which I filed myself. The countless needless hardships that befell city hospital patients daily, that any intern or resident could recite off the top of his head, either proved too commonplace or too threatening to the average house officer for him to document. The result was the eventual abandonment of the project and the demise of our formal CIR efforts in the area of patient care.

I finished my tenure as CIR president in a dour and discouraged frame of mind. Dimmer's words about the untrustworthiness of physicians echoed in my ears and I felt then—as I do *not* now—that house staff were hopelessly bourgeois and useless as a force for change in the medical-care system. In my glum moments I chose to ignore a number of significant developments that were taking place around me. During my time with the CIR an executive assistant had been hired who worked full time for the organization, getting its finances together. More important, she began a four-page newspaper—*The CIR Reports*—which appeared every six weeks or so. Many of us wrote for it, covering topics ranging from reports on contract negotiations to muckraking on hospital conditions. Generally it gave interns and residents a sense of being part of a system rather than merely a member of a department or a doctor at an isolated hospital. Even if our two-pronged attack had not proven it, interest in the system and the politics of the system was growing rapidly. In subsequent years the CIR would develop a full-time central staff including a young lawyer hired to assist Murray Gordon for CIR affairs exclusively. A number of physicians would take time off during or after their training to work as organizers for the CIR, something unheard of in previous years. And the membership—now increasingly involved in the organization —paid for all this by voting dues increases on themselves.

Interest in house staff organizing was by no means limited to New York. A group of us committed to seeing the idea grow convened the first Assembly of House Staff Organizations in St. Louis in the winter of 1971. Several hundred house officers from around the nation showed up. There were, to be sure, many differences among the young doctors: big hospital *vs.* small hospital; political experience and achievement *vs.* fear of the administration and job reprisals; pro-union, labor mentality *vs.* anti-union convictions. But the majority of those who attended had more in common than not and a steering committee managed to hang together and organize a second and then a third conference in subsequent years before the Physicians' National House Staff Association (PNHA) was born. Several years later the PNHA is thriving, winning benefits for its members and generally making a name for younger physicians by taking progressive stands on health-care issues and battling the AMA on numerous questions.

The CIR has become much more activist in recent years. The house officers themselves have been clear that at this point they are not looking for higher salaries but want to see some sort of ceiling put on their work load—both for their benefit and for the well-being of their patients. In the winter of 1975 the CIR went on strike—a new experience for the CIR, New York, and the nation. The issue was the right to *discuss* hours on duty in the contract negotiation and the target was not, in fact, the city hospitals (the city agreed to negotiate hours) but the affiliated private hospitals with which the CIR also held contracts. The League of Voluntary Hospitals, representing these institutions, refused to discuss schedules. They held that the chief of each service should continue to set work hours as he saw fit. The CIR said no and, after negotiations failed, they threw up picket lines around the institutions and went public. The press supported the doctors' action. Why, they wanted to know, were the hospitals afraid to discuss an eighty-hour week, or even a hundred-hour week? Surely they would want such precautions for their patients. Work in excess of those figures could not be considered valuable or safe, they reasoned. By the end of a week the League agreed to the establishment of committees in each hospital to review and define work hours on a department-by-department basis. The committees were defined and guaranteed in the CIR contract. The interns and residents went back to work newly confident of their own muscle. Their action, though, had done much more than simply win them fewer hours on the job. The reasonable use of house officers which will come in the wake of the CIR victory will cause a whole series of staffing reforms that will improve patient care immensely. By fighting and winning on a "self-interest" issue the CIR will have done a great deal for hospital reform.

In my time with the CIR I would never have believed such a strategy could have worked. I believed then in "new waves" and militant, direct idealism. I would have predicted then that the seventies would prove a time of increasing house staff influence and the expression of generally liberal or radical political tendencies by younger physicians. That has, in large part, come to pass but not at all in the manner I envisioned. The developments have come about more as a quiet, continuous ripple than as a wave. The philosophy governing the effort comes not from the SDS or the SHO but from a blend of sound labor practice, liberal politics, and an agonizing first-hand familiarity with the crisis state of our medical care system. That amalgam of experience sets the current intern or resident apart from his predecessors in a significant way. Moreover, it appears durable and suggests the development of what we always hoped for—a new and progressive focus for younger physicians bent on changing and improving the role of the medical profession in America.

5

The Lincoln Project

The single issue that united and motivated politically active interns and residents more than any other was community involvement in medical centers. The situation at Jacobi was typical. Like almost all teaching hospitals, it lacked any sense of community base or any vehicle for community input. Jacobi had no community board, no patient advocates, no ombudsman, and no avenue of community redress or review. The administration was accountable to the City Department of Hospitals and to the medical school. That was all. This, though, was after five years of major urban upheaval in the United States when communities—especially poor and oppressed communities —had expressed their anger at being taken for granted. More important, the Oceanhill–Brownsville battle over community control of schools had already taken place, signaling a coherent and legalistic assault by minority communities on city government for control of services in their areas. Yet Jacobi, like her kindred academic hospitals around the country, showed no inclination to move toward any form of community input.

We believed strongly in the SDS maxim of "participatory democracy." This had been a guiding principle of the SHO and we all carried it with us as we became workers in medical facilities. It meant simply that the people served by an institution should have a major say about the policies and the directions of that institution. If they do not, the priorities established will be those of some other group who may or may not be well intentioned and who may or may not be sensitive and wise to the needs of the people to be served. The people themselves will have been disenfranchised with respect to that institution: the quality, style, and even the existence of those services will be out of their hands. In poor urban neighborhoods this disenfranchisement is often complete; what matters a single vote every few years when the hospitals, schools, garbage, street security, bus routes, and even heroin traffic are determined by men who at best know only the statistics of the neighborhood and, more often than not, make their decisions in terms of their own power rather than community needs.

We did not want to become the enforcers of such a system: the angry white cop on the beat in the black neighborhood; the frustrated middle-class teacher in the Spanish-speaking classroom; the infuriated fireman ducking bricks as he tries to hose down burning mattresses in a vacant lot. We did not want to become the medical analogue of these executors of the urban system.

Yet our training program and the style of medicine we practiced invited it. We treated patients who came from New York's various ethnic neighborhoods with absolutely no reference to their backgrounds, their expectations, or their medical beliefs. We were an anonymous corps of white-coated physicians dispensing our medicines, in our hospital, on our terms, with little or no information about the communities or people we processed. The majority of our patients were distinctly ethnic (black, Puerto Rican, Italian, and Jewish) with customs and beliefs that undoubtedly bore on their care. We made no home visits, worked with no community organizations, visited no local practitioners, and generally maintained a kind of medical school isolation despite the fact that we were a city hospital. We were faithful to academic teachings and the most current medical literature, but we hardly knew our patients.

Working the Emergency Room one night I entered a cubicle to find a Puerto Rican child wheezing loudly and uncomfortably with asthma. His young mother fanned him with a newspaper. I asked her to remove his shirt so I could listen with a stethoscope. When she did I discovered his chest was cross-hatched with a pink clay-like substance. I suppose I looked perplexed because the mother became embarrassed and covered his chest quickly with the shirt. It was nothing, she said, just a home remedy. I tried to minimize my curiosity and started my therapy for asthma. As the boy's condition improved and the mother began to relax I asked her again about the marks on his chest. She bowed her head and fumbled with the newspaper for a moment and then said, "It wasn't my idea. It was my mother's. She still believes in *Botanicas*. I told her it wouldn't work but she wouldn't listen to me. She said we should try it first because it was the old way and the good way. So we took him and they tried many cures including the marks on the chest. But he just got worse so I rushed him over here. I didn't have time to wash his chest. I'm sorry." I knew only that *Botanicas* could be found on street corners in many neighborhoods in the Bronx and that they were centers for the practice of Puerto Rican folk medicine. How many of my patients used them before, during, or after my therapy I have no idea. More, probably, than I would have guessed.

My successful treatment of the youth's asthma did not prove the superiority of "Western" medicine over Caribbean folk craft. Rather it underscored my ignorance of the people and the community I purported to serve. In the same manner that the hospital declined to recognize the community politically, my training program (like others throughout the country) did not acknowledge the community medically. Neither were we told about the significance of the community in general nor were we encouraged to learn its style and idiosyncrasies in particular.

The result of the categorical isolation of the medical center from the community was not simply unrest on the part of a few of us who thought this wrong. The real outcome is what both physicians and patients have come to know as "city hospital care" or "teaching hospital care." Impersonal, unpredictable, marked by long waits, rarely administered by the same physician on successive visits, "city hospital medicine" is nobody's ideal of good or sensitive medical care. Because out-patient clinics, emergency rooms, and teaching hospital wards are staffed by an endless rotation of house officers of varying skills, it is pure chance which physician sees which patient for which illness at a given time. If the illness requires repeated emergency room or out-patient visits, the patient is *likely* to see a different doctor on each trip. Ironically, the worse or, particularly, the more esoteric the disease, the less likely the patient is to suffer the full impact of the impersonality of the system. An unfortunate individual with leukemia, for example, or an itinerant arriving with malaria can count on seeing the professor of hematology on each visit. The unusual nature of the disease and its "teaching value" will assure far better continuity for that patient than for the unhappy mother of a two-year-old with repeated respiratory infections or the adult with chronic stomach pain from a low-grade ulcer. These unlucky patients will be bumped and shuttled around the system indefinitely. To the extent that continuity of care and warm, trusting human contact are important in the practice of "Western" medicine, they will not find them in the teaching hospital system.

Then, too, we objected to the blanket presumption that all of us were going into private practice. Since an overwhelming majority of America's physicians are private practitioners, the expectation that most of us were bound toward the lucrative land of fee-for-service medicine was not an unreasonable one. Yet it irked many of us who believed there should be and, to a very real extent were, alternatives to private practice. The continual reference to private medicine not only annoyed us but it came across as a statement of political support for the present dual system of medical care in the United States. "When you're out on your own in private practice," our attendings (many of whom were themselves private practitioners) would often say, "and you see a patient with such and such disease, you will . . ." Or again, "When you're treating your private patients with such and such condition, you should . . ." And, most insultingly, "You can't expect patients here [city hospital] to understand, but when you're treating your own patients, you ought to explain . . ."

Private medicine, the allusions seemed to say, is good medicine, real medicine. The city hospital or the teaching hospital is just a warm-up, the proving grounds, the dummy scrimmage. Behind those statements lay a tacit understanding: there *are* two systems of medical care in the United States and they are quite obviously unequal. There is the private system for the well-to-do, the insured, the fully employed, and many more who struggle to hold on against heavy financial odds. And then there is the other system—the public system, the charity system, the city system. It travels by many names but, ironically, it is more nearly a true system than the private system because its style and quality are predictable throughout the country. It is a system for the poor and those whom social scientists choose to call the "medically indigent," who may not be really poor but can't afford what private medicine costs. It is, simply, a separate and unequal second-class system.

That physicians acknowledged the bipartite nature of American medical care, that many medical schools chose to live comfortably off the resultant inequities, making the hospitals for the poor their "teaching" hospitals, struck us as cynical in the extreme. What rankled me most about the continuous presumption that I intended to become a private practitioner after my city hospital tenure was that it not only assumed that I would be happy to abandon the care of the poor but that it expected me to embrace the hypocrisy of the dual system.

That was not the route I wanted or expected to go and I knew that many young medical workers shared those sentiments. The medical school with its liberal appearance, its intellectual base, and its apparent effort to deal with the medical problems of the poor held an appeal for me. Given the circumstances, especially given private practice as the major alternative, the medical school avenue looked good. But in truth, the medical school was every bit as wed to the system as were the private practitioners. Two years working at Jacobi, Einstein's primary teaching hospital, had taught me that.

Reflecting on the paradoxes of medical school medical care, I was reminded of a debate that has occurred over the past few years concerning an eminent American medical researcher. Virologist, pediatrician, department chairman, he has performed outstanding and extremely practical investigations on hepatitis, an infection that has been little understood until recently and for which we have no cure. Using severely retarded children at a state-run home for the care of mental defectives, he has systematically studied the disease by feeding new arrivals small quantities of hepatitis-infected stool. Under these "well-controlled" circumstances he has been able to separate two different types of hepatitis, characterize their course, and begin to develop vaccines against them.

But what of the children fed hepatitis as orientation to their new home? Numerous critics have challenged the ethics of the research, decrying the use of essentially defenseless retardates in potentially dangerous experiments for the betterment of the rest of society. The researcher, however, defends his work neither in terms of medical innocuousness (he admits that hepatitis is a dangerous illness to contract) nor in terms of social utility (the society is more important than the individual so these retardates must be risked), but in terms of a grim pragmatism. In the institution for the retarded, hepatitis is rampant, he notes. Virtually every inmate contracts it sooner or later. His administration of the disease under controlled circumstances, therefore, is not unscrupulous but merely a scientific variation on what would happen anyway. This indeed is an accurate marshaling of the facts about these children and their institution. This practical argument blunts much of the criticism of his research. Yet it ignores, it comfortably forgets the much larger and more compelling conclusion about the care of the retarded. Their institution is so overcrowded and so poorly staffed that stool contamination—circulating shit—is ever-present and guaranteed to transmit hepatitis and a variety of other stool-borne diseases to every resident. The researcher, his team, his department, and his university choose not to challenge the circumstances of life at the hospital but rather accept them and live comfortably off them. Public health issues and state hospital budgets are not their concern, they would argue. They are virologists. Their job is the pursuit of the truth about hepatitis. It is for others to change the institutions.

The self-interested aloofness of this example parallels the situation with medical schools which live quite respectably off city and county hospitals whose level of care they officially find reprehensible but whose wards they happily fill with eager students, interns, and residents who treat patients with no choice but to accept what care they get. The schools are wed to poverty medicine as the researcher is beholden to freely circulating stool.

Marty Stein was a good and old friend. Son of a Los Angeles shopkeeper, graduate of Berkeley in the days of the Free Speech Movement, and partisan of the SHO, he came to Jacobi at the same time I did. During long nights on duty or at quiet moments in the Emergency Room, we debated many of these points. We were learning a lot of medicine. We knew that. But weren't we becoming an indistinguishable part of the system? We had been involved in the Jacobi "actions" (the sixteen-dollar fee fight and the battle over the budget cuts) but increasingly they seemed to us isolated and limited events. They had had little real or permanent impact on the hospital and less on the system as a whole. And where were we headed personally? We were rapidly completing our second year of pediatric training, a milestone on the road to Pediatric Specialty Boards. But what of our earlier commitment to social change and medical progressivism?

We discovered that we shared a sense of isolation. There were many people at Jacobi whom we liked and even a reasonable number with whom we felt close politically. But we and our political friends were in a tiny minority. By everybody's admission the agenda of Jacobi was medical education, medical research, and city-style medical care for the large numbers of people who arrived daily at the hospital expecting help. Given the size of Jacobi and the clarity of its mission in the eyes of those supporting it, it seemed far-fetched indeed that a handful of us could stand up and say, "Hold everything! Can't you see that what we're doing here supports the continuation of bad medical care? Can't you understand that our practice of medicine under these circumstances insults and oppresses communities of people we purport to serve and who need our respect and support badly?"

We laughed at the absurdity of the thought, but Marty came up with an idea that made a great deal of sense and started our thinking in an entirely new direction. He talked of a *critical mass*, a concept borrowed from physics to describe the amount of activated material necessary to produce a chain reaction in a much larger quantity of previously inert matter. "We need to be in a setting with enough like-minded people who object to the present way of practicing medicine so that ideas can grow and have impact." We knew in fact that there were many residents, interns, and senior medical students who shared our perspective but, having no alternative, had spread themselves around the country in a variety of traditional programs where their complaints, like ours, were easily absorbed. The SHO, which still functioned in some areas, and our contacts with old SHO members could provide us with an instant roster of potential recruits for a radical, community-oriented internship-residency program.

Our enthusiasm grew as we talked. We were joined in our discussions by Barbara Blase, a fellow resident who had been involved in the Jacobi actions with us. We had all complained at one time or another about the lack of relevant training programs. There seemed to be no politically consistent bridge between the principles we developed in medical school and the kind of medicine we hoped to practice after our period of training. Now, though, Marty, Barbara, and I had a cogent recruitment plan for staffing such a program.

But where could it happen? Jacobi, a 1,200-bed hospital, already had almost 400 interns and residents and a clearly defined purpose which did not include experiments in institutional control or community relations. Moreover, no matter how successful our recruitment plans, we would be swallowed by the sheer size of Jacobi. For our critical mass to be truly critical, the setting would have to be small and, preferably, much more closely identified with a given neighborhood than a referral center like Jacobi.

It didn't take us long to think of the place. We all knew Lincoln Hospital, a small, ancient, dilapidated city hospital in the South Bronx, serving one of New York's most oppressed neighborhoods. It was a poor-sister affiliate of Einstein College of Medicine, and we all rotated there for one or two months a year. Curiously, in spite of Lincoln's nineteenth-century plant, its battle-zone mentality, and its cockroach-infested on-call rooms, the place had a hold on us even before we considered going there full time. We liked it. There was an immediacy, a relevancy, a passion to the medical life at Lincoln, and the staff—medical and nonmedical—seemed to sense it. And Lincoln's community was in no way a theoretical concept. Day and night, week and weekend, the people came. They arrived from the adjacent streets, walking with their children or traveling a few stops on the bus or subway. For the most part, they were black or Puerto Rican but, like the white immigrants who had occupied the neighborhood before them, many called the hospital the Butcher Shop.

We had no notion at that time of Lincoln's antebellum origins as a home for freed slaves nor of its century and a half of life in the best and most paradoxical traditions of American racism. Neither did we have any idea of the eventual political reverberations that would develop around our nascent scheme for a new model medical training program. But Lincoln met all the criteria Marty and I had worked out for a hospital with a small medical staff, a real community base, a medical school affiliation necessary for the training program and, additionally, a chronic problem of understaffing. We decided to pursue our idea by talking with some friends who were already working full time at Lincoln.

The Pediatric Department at Lincoln consisted almost entirely of foreign-trained physicians. No different from many other city and small private "community" hospitals, this situation arises out of the inequities of the American medical system. At present rates we graduate annually only about half the number of medical students that we need to fill the intern and resident positions we have open. Academically this matters little, but from a service standpoint it leaves a mammoth gap in our primary line of medical defense. Many city and community hospitals have never recruited an American-trained graduate to cover their house physician responsibilities. Without a steady stream of foreign-trained applicants, there might well have been medical manpower crises in all of these areas long before the present. These crises most likely would have produced the demand for the education of more American physicians or the training of community people for a variety of intermediate skills, such as Emergency Room technicians, midwives, and pediatric associates, to relieve the shortage of doctors. The demand has never really developed, however, because there has been an ever-present pool of young physicians trained in the Philippines, India, Pakistan, the Dominican Republic, Thailand, and elsewhere. One-third of the medical licenses issued in the United States each year go to foreign medical graduates, and the number of foreign-trained physicians that enter this country annually now exceeds the number of Americans we graduate from medical school.

These figures described an unfortunate tariff placed on certain small nations by a rich one. The physicians come in search of medical education but also seeking the American way of life. They find both (the latter more consistently than the former) and often they stay. The more ambitious are not satisfied with the absence of real teaching at most small private hospitals and gravitate toward the cities and teaching centers, hoping to get a break and find their way into the mainstream of American medicine. Lincoln, rough and bedraggled but affiliated with a medical school, consistently attracted many good foreign-trained physicians.

In 1970 all but two of the pediatric house staff were foreign trained. The two, Charlotte Phillips and David Stead, had chosen Lincoln on principle. Both could easily have found more prestigious jobs at better-recognized teaching centers. Yet both decided to do their internship and residency at Lincoln because it was a community-based hospital relatively free of the trappings of medical school protocol and hierarchy. Charlotte was a veteran of student political activity, working as an early SDS member at Swarthmore and later participating in the founding of the SHO in Cleveland. She had lived for several years during medical school in a slum neighborhood participating in local political organizing. When she came to New York she visited Jacobi and surely would have been added to the staff if she had wanted to be. But the academic hustle-bustle of the place and the clear (clearer to her than to me) absence of a community base in our program turned her off. Instead she decided to accept a position at Lincoln. I remember being nonplused at the idea. Why had she turned down a chance to work with Marty and me and our other political house staff in a prestigious—if alienating—setting to go to a rundown, overwhelmed hospital nobody had ever heard of? In retrospect, I realize that she understood a lot about the work place that I was not to appreciate for some time and she sensed a difference in the two institutions that took me two years to discover.

Marty, Barbara, and I approached Charlotte and David with our idea for what we came to call the "Lincoln Project." They liked it immediately. While neither of them had gone to Lincoln as a self-conscious "first wave" of a new program, both felt isolated. They served their patients, learned pediatrics, and did the best they could medically. But they lacked allies and found no real interest in political issues among the other house staff. The foreign graduates were at Lincoln, simply enough, to learn medicine. The details of American medical care and health rights were of no interest to them. Understandably, the notion that we would recruit others with a political interest in changing health care to join them on the staff at Lincoln appealed to Charlotte and David. After discussing the idea in broad terms, we agreed to a division of labor. No one had spoken to any of the powers within the Department of Pediatrics where we were plotting our recruitment drive. David and Charlotte would speak to Dr. Arnold Einhorn, the director of pediatrics at Lincoln, their immediate boss, while Marty, Barbara, and I would talk to the chairman of pediatrics at Einstein in whose domain Lincoln fell. Without the blessings of both the pope and the archbishop, as we playfully dubbed the pediatric potentates, our plan could go nowhere.

The task that Marty, Barbara, and I took on proved an easy one, Dr. Henry Barnett, the department chairman, and his assistant, Dr. Lewis Fraad, approved the idea immediately. Barnett, an eminent nephrologist and something of a pediatric statesman, and Fraad, a veteran backer of progressive innovation in medicine, had both supported the SHO in its prime and knew of our restiveness at Jacobi. Welcoming our sense of experimentation, approving its general direction, and, perhaps, privately delighted that it was to take place in someone else's bailiwick, they wished us well in our project. They agreed to assist us by supplying the names and addresses of all the applicants to the Jacobi pediatric program so that we might get in touch with them to publicize our program. Finally they admonished us to discuss things slowly and carefully with Dr. Einhorn, whose department we proposed to renovate. They dared not predict his reaction but without his approval, they reminded us, the program could go nowhere. This warning proved far more prophetic than we and, I suspect, they realized at the time.

In 1970 Arnold Einhorn was in his mid-40s. A full professor of pediatrics at Einstein, co-author with Dr. Barnett of one of America's outstanding pediatric textbooks, answerable only to Dr. Barnett at Einstein and accountable, really, to no one at Lincoln, he ran his department with an authoritarian hand. As a youth during the Second World War, Dr. Einhorn had been imprisoned in France because of his Belgian Jewish ancestry. He escaped, made his way across the Pyrenees to Spain, and from there found his way to Palestine. He returned to France at the end of the war and settled down to study medicine. In the early fifties he came to the United States to complete his medical training. He applied at the newly formed Einstein–Jacobi complex but was referred to the ever-available Lincoln to serve a year's novitiate. Lincoln in the early fifties was at its all-time low. The hospital lacked both staff and budget and, the story goes, everybody did everything—that is, everything they could. Einhorn never talked much about the experience except to say that there were five residents to do what we were recruiting thirty-five to handle.

He served well and graduated to Jacobi where he became a resident and a chief resident of exceptional abilities. On finishing his house officership he elected to stay on in academic medicine, but in spite of his clear skills as a physician and teacher he could not be characterized as a diplomat. The same compulsiveness and precision that made him an exacting clinician, and that we were to observe almost two decades later, made him a difficult man to work with. Early on it was suggested that he return to Lincoln, remaining an integral part of the Pediatric Department of Einstein, and attempt to build a first-rate teaching service out of the rubble of a woefully neglected city hospital. He accepted.

From the late fifties on, long before any other department at Einstein formally affiliated with Lincoln and many years in advance of the now popular affiliations between other New York medical schools and city hospitals, Einhorn labored at Lincoln. Starting with a tiny house staff, few other attending physicians, minimal nursing, a decrepit plant and a penny-ante budget, Einhorn began to build *his* department. Gradually things improved. By the mid-sixties the affiliation concept had come into its own accompanied by increased budget and recognition. Einhorn's meticulous attention to every detail of teaching and patient care overcame many of the obstacles of city hospital medicine and his service gained sufficient reputation so that recruitment of house staff—foreign house staff—ceased to be a major problem. This meant, for instance, that Lincoln Pediatrics could fill its openings from foreign medical graduates who had already spent a year or more in this country, insuring a certain facility with the language and, ideally, letters of reference from directors of training programs here. Under Einhorn's tutelage, the quality of physician and of medical care in Lincoln Pediatrics improved immensely.

During these years Einhorn's prowess as a clinician and a teacher continued to grow. To be sure, he was rarely surrounded by medical equals, but he read the literature avidly, contributed to it occasionally, and examined personally virtually every child with a major or interesting ailment who passed through Lincoln during a fifteen-year period. There was not an unusual medical condition of which he had not seen one or, perhaps, a dozen examples. He became a professor in the European tradition, revered and feared by his students, armed with an anecdote for every illness, unequaled as a diagnostician but also unchallenged in his diagnoses. He developed a protocol or a system for everything from the treatment of the adrenogenital syndrome to the recording of unusual cases (the notorious "IPF" or Interesting Patient File). His mandates were followed slavishly by residents who not infrequently executed treatment plans for a single reason—because Dr. Einhorn said to.

Over the years Einhorn performed a Herculean feat for which I respect him medically and, I cannot deny it, politically. While several generations of physicians sought and found lucrative jobs in private practice or prestigious jobs in medical schools, Arnold Einhorn devoted himself doggedly to the care of the children of one of America's worst slums, and the medical education of several hundred young physicians from all corners of the world. Subsequent events cannot deny him that monumental achievement. But Einhorn became virtually unchallenged ruler of his tiny feifdom. His residents did not stay in his department to help him build it. Class after class completed their training and left Lincoln and the South Bronx as well. The senior physicians he chose to staff the department generally offered little challenge to the professor. Most pediatricians of promise or ambition who did become part of the staff over the years usually found Einhorn's attentiveness and omnipresence insufferable and passed on quickly. The result was that the Lincoln Pediatric Department *was* Arnold Einhorn. The house staff knew it, the few attendings gathered around him knew it and, most significantly, Einhorn knew it.

It fell to Charlotte and David to approach this skilled and difficult man with our plan for a new house staff for his department. Gamely they outlined our idea to him not at all knowing what response to expect. He indicated interest in the proposal and asked that the five of us—Marty, Barbara, and me included—sit down with him to review the idea.

We met late one afternoon at his Lincoln office, a smallish, dark room lined with pediatrics texts, a modest and functional base for a department director. A short man with an amiable face, clad, as always, in a knee-length white coat, he chatted comfortably with us. He spoke with a trace of a French accent. Much to our surprise, he listened only briefly to our outline and then stated unequivocal support for the program. "I have worked here at Lincoln for many years in the hope of improving medical care for the poor. Finally there seems to be someone else who agrees with me. The people uptown (meaning the medical school) pay a lot of lip service to the idea but they don't do much about it. I think your idea sounds like a good one. Where do we begin?"

In fact the only negative note in the whole discussion was his warning to deal with him and not "the people uptown." He knew that we had approached Barnett and Fraad before we talked to him and that angered him. "This is my department," he told us in tones we would hear again, "and I'll run it. Do business with me and we'll get along fine."

Surprised but pleased that Einhorn had embraced our plan so readily, we debated among ourselves what could have been the reason. We had outlined the idea only in rather vague terms, since our own thinking was still fairly vague. We had promised to recruit American-trained interns and residents interested in community medicine to staff the department. They would perform the traditional duties of house officers but would have several months a year of "community elective." (All medical training programs feature elective time when the young physician can choose to concentrate more intensely in an area of special interest—traditionally cardiology, hematology, or the like. We proposed that interns and residents in our program spend the time in the community working with community organizations or political groups.) Additionally we suggested the establishment of "continuity clinics" where all house officers would care for patients long term in an effort to combat city hospital impersonality and discontinuity.

Einhorn greeted all these suggestions with enthusiasm. It seemed clear to us, though he never said it, that most important of all to this seasoned teacher of doctors was our promise of an American house staff. Foreign-trained as he was, Einhorn certainly had sympathy and understanding for the plight of non-American physicians in the United States. Yet the goal, the medical status symbol, of an American house staff for *his* program had eluded him through the years. At last, it must have seemed, the value of his work and his pedagogy had been recognized, and graduates of America's most prestigious medical schools were beginning to come to him to be trained as pediatricians. Surely and understandably that belief was attractive and gratifying to the veteran pediatrician.

In talking with Einhorn about our plan, we mentioned one further point which passed without much discussion; perhaps because it was less concrete and apparently more philosophical it invited no immediate attention on his part. We talked of involving the community in the department to a greater degree. To us this meant working out a scheme for community input, some measure of community control. It is hard to know what it meant to Einhorn. Most likely it suggested increased ties with community agencies and more aggressive efforts at community health education. Certainly he never intended to share the reins of his department with anyone and he surely did not take our proposal to mean that. However, the issue passed undisputed. The degree to which he had accepted our plan so stunned us that it seemed picayune to pursue a "what if . . ." theoretical debate at that point. The accord was so overwhelming that our task seemed to be to get to work and not pause for further definitions. Neither we nor the department director had any notion at that first meeting how far apart our thinking really was on the key question of the validity and importance of the community vis-à-vis the hospital. Moreover, none of us could have known then how precipitously events would move in the ensuing months to make our discord clearly and painfully apparent.

We went busily to work. With some thirty intern and resident positions to fill, recruitment obviously became the first order of business. Meeting weekly with Einhorn to review the responses received, the community organizations contacted, the program planning carried out, we slowly assembled a roster of young physicians prepared to come to Lincoln on July 1, 1970 to begin work as part of a Community Pediatrics Program. Interest in the program ran high. Using old SHO contacts for the most part, we scoured the country for senior medical students, interns, and residents willing to try an experiment in medical education and patient care. Many responded favorably and selection among the hopefuls proved to be more of a problem than generating interest. The new applications, many from people we knew, were discussed in detail with Einhorn and acted on by him with our advice. The process was both cordial and exciting. In the end we recruited eighteen interns, five first-year residents, and six second-year residents—a successful job by any standards.

We agreed with Einhorn that preference should be given to the members of the then current Lincoln pediatric staff who wanted to stay for the new program. The director would invite those interns and residents he wanted to remain as part of the department. In the end some ten stayed, predominantly Filipinos, equally divided between men and women. Relations among Charlotte, David, Marty, myself, and these Lincoln residents were generally warm. We had all worked together for varying periods of time at Lincoln; we trusted and enjoyed each other. But as the new program took shape a subtle schism began to form between the old residents and the incoming group. We were coming to Lincoln with political as well as personal and medical goals, whereas they were staying on for the same reasons they had come in the first place—medical training they could not obtain in their own countries. Moreover, they were deeply indebted to Dr. Einhorn. Not only had he selected them in the first place but he had singled them out as the best of his staff and asked them to stay for the new program. They had an allegiance to the department director shared by none of the new house staff who had selected Lincoln often knowing nothing of Einhorn. The American graduates came to Lincoln beholden to one another and not to the department or its director. This was a new circumstance in the Pediatric Department and one that would become more obvious and more troublesome in time.

Many of the recruits came from the New York area. Both the heavy concentration of medical schools in the region and the greater ease with which we could contact New York people dictated that. As more people became interested and committed we began to have biweekly and then weekly meetings of what we still called the Lincoln Project. The meetings served to keep everyone informed of progress and also to assign recruitment and publicity tasks to individuals and committees.

Over the course of the meetings an increasingly coherent philosophical and political position emerged. First of all our new program would be committed to service. We all shared the criticism of teaching hospitals and medicine in general that frequently patient care is obstructed by hidden agendas of the providers of care—research, teaching, and money. We intended to dedicate our program to good patient service despite the obstacles. Second, we were interested in what we called "community control." The patient—the consumer—had been excluded too long from having a say in his own medical care and we saw it as our job to build bridges, to form alliances with community groups who could begin to participate actively in the affairs of the hospital. And finally we agreed on collectivism as our mode of operation. The notion of collectivism was extremely popular among student groups and progressive organizations at the time. The idea implied absolute democracy among participants in a group without the traditional emergence of leadership and hierarchy. Decisions would be made by the group as a group. Criticism and support would be freely exchanged among group members in an effort to develop all of the members together and discourage individuals from using the group for personal or self-serving ends. In recognition of these ideals we began formally to call ourselves the Pediatric Collective.

Late in the spring of 1970 we held the first meeting of the entire group committed to start on July first. The get-together took place on a May weekend in the shabby auditorium of the Lincoln Nurses' Residence, a building adjacent to the hospital, once used to house the Lincoln School for Nurses. We pooled funds to meet the cost of plane tickets for people from outside the New York area. It was a heady feeling when we all came together for the first time, the first flush of collectivism, the first real sense that the idea talked about for so long was being realized. The style and sense of the gathering was more that of a folk concert than a medical convocation. Sandals and beards were prominent. Counting the wives, nurses, and friends present, women easily outnumbered the men. People greeted one another with embraces as often as not. Political literature circulated. There was an intensity to the entire experience. These were people who had come together to discuss more than a job, a training program, a medical experience. People had come to Lincoln to share their politics, to join their lives, to work together. The meeting reflected that.

But the meeting also supplied us with our first taste of acrimony and division. Things did not go well with Einhorn. Joining us the first morning, he welcomed newcomers and told them he was excited about the new program. A debate developed quickly, however, about the nature of community elective. The New York City Department of Health had been in touch with Dr. Einhorn, offering to turn over a Well Baby Station (a city facility for newborn exams and baby shots) to the Department of Pediatrics for our program. We would provide rotating physicians, presumably on community elective, to staff the facility and the city would supply nurses, medications, and the site. We could run it in any way we liked doing outreach, health education, community organizing, and so forth. To Einhorn it seemed like a good opportunity and well within his definition of community activity. Some of the Collective agreed but the majority felt that community elective should be used for something more radical (people talked vaguely of staffing Black Panther clinics or doing health organizing for local political groups). Anyway, they argued, we would be doing the city's work for them (rather than pushing them to do it themselves) and we would subject ourselves to ultimate control and cooptation by the Department of Health. The offer was voted down, beginning a protracted battle between Einhorn and the Collective as to what community elective should really be.

Generally we spent the weekend raising issues rather than resolving them. But that was in the nature of our undertaking. Never had a house staff added a political element to their medical training nor had a house staff ever organized its own program from scratch. The topics we discussed were both traditional and highly nontraditional. We covered rotations, amounts of elective time, night-call schedule, and teaching responsibilities. We also debated salary sharing, communal living, and our common politics. The latter issues proved far more difficult than the former. Most people felt that we should pool some of our individual salaries to use for support of community groups and actions that were in need of financial help. The sticky question, though, was whether the money should be voluntarily donated or whether the Collective should set a tithe on everybody's income. At length the topic was tabled. The housing question solved itself more easily. A number of Collective members agreed to find a house together close to Lincoln and share living expenses. Subsequently several other Lincoln groups did likewise.

Despite the common background of many of the Collective members and despite the parallel sentiments that had brought us to Lincoln, it turned out to be extremely difficult to define our politics. Clearly our style and our roots were New Left rather than Old Left. Our politics were not so much learned as they were felt. With us, as with the New Left in general, the term "politics" assumed moral connotations. Politics meant neither an electoral process nor a party allegiance but referred to one's stance toward the system. Someone who was political or who practiced "good" politics was someone who stood in a position of challenge or resistance to oppressive or corrupt elements of the political and economic systems that related to themselves and the people they worked with. Someone whose politics were "bad" was someone who used the system for personal gain, usually at the expense of others. If they tended toward the moralistic and judgmental, our political sentiments were, nevertheless, honest, heartfelt, and functional.

On the other hand, we were not at all well read or well schooled in the thinking of the Left. Few of us had actually studied Marx, Lenin, Trotsky, or even Marcuse or Regis Debray. Aside from college survey courses, most of us were ignorant of economics and history. Generally we lacked the perspective and discipline that characterized the Old Left. Becoming politicized in medical school as most of us had, reacting to inequities we had seen there, we were well versed in academic brawls and departmental infighting, but we knew little about trade unionism and less about American socialism. Our class background differed little from that of any group of young physicians. We had not succeeded in recruiting any Puerto Ricans or blacks for the program.

Subjective, then, as we were in our approach to politics, I think we shared some basically sound instincts. Radicalism was the object of "good" politics. To be radical meant, literally, to go to the root of the problem and look for solutions there, rather than to be satisfied with partial or self-serving answers. Honestly and reasonably we considered ourselves radicals. Beyond that we found absolute definitions of our politics elusive. Again we tabled the debate with, I think, more accord than we felt.

Women played a major role in the style and dynamics of the Collective from the first weekend meeting. Almost a third of the physicians in the Collective were women. Additionally, a number of nurses and many wives attended the organizational Collective meeting. They formed a women's caucus and resolved to continue to meet as a women's group to discuss problems relevant to Lincoln and to themselves as women. The impact of their self-consciousness and their organizational activity was to help shape the Collective in the months to come.

Significantly the community too came to the first meeting. The South Bronx, the vaguely defined southern extremity of New York's largest (geographically) borough, is home for more than 300,000 people. Set against that magnitude and density of population the term community withers. Who are legitimate representatives of the community? Block clubs, boys clubs, church groups, the borough president, political bosses, street gangs? We had obvious prejudices as to those we thought had the best claim to representing the community. In such an uncharted and, ultimately, competitive situation, choices were mandatory. Our selection ran toward those who were activist, angry, and, most important, those who were interested in basic social change rather than patronage or profit. Speaking practically, we were interested in people who were interested in Lincoln. Several groups had already been active in and around the hospital and their representatives volunteered to join us in our planning sessions. The Black Panther party and the Young Lord party, both of whom were working in the South Bronx at the time, were there. The most significant input came from several workers from the Lincoln Community Mental Health Service. Members of the neighborhood and employees of the hospital, they instructed the Collective in the recent political history of the hospital and the area.

Later Einhorn and others would argue that we chose to align ourselves with "radicals" and "militants" from the start. I cannot disagree with this analysis though I by no means accept it as a derogatory commentary on the Collective. Our interest, indeed our purpose, in being at Lincoln was in seeing medical care in the hospital and in the community improve and improve rapidly. There were many groups in and around the hospital—the medical school, the Medical Board of the hospital, the official Community Board of the hospital, to mention a few—who had programs that called for more or less the same changes. Yet each of these groups had other agendas that either obscured or obliterated any possibility of that change. In every instance, the status quo had too much to offer in the way of money, position, or power to risk any basic innovation. The "radicals" we chose to associate with were not without agendas or ambitions of their own, but they were not in business for self-aggrandizement. Their view of health was part of their broader notion of community and human development. A hospital was not a mere pawn in the intrigues of ghetto politics. It was, rather, a living institution that could and should express the best and the most humane side of societal life. Their actions were predicated on that view and for that they were called radical. We happily joined them in accepting the epithet.

The first Collective meeting ended well enough. To be sure there had been disagreement both within and without the Collective but there had also been a great deal of accord, warmth, and excitement. We could all see the idea taking form, coming to life, enveloping us. What were a few arguments among ourselves or a disagreement with Einhorn when we had thirty friends coming together to do an important job, a job that needed doing, a job that could influence the way others learned and practiced medicine around the country?

We looked forward to July First with anticipation.

6

The Butcher Shop

Working at Lincoln was a new sort of experience for me as for other members of the Collective. As students, interns, and residents we had all seen a variety of hospitals. We were all versed in—even hardened to—the private hospital/city hospital dichotomy. But Lincoln was not just another city hospital. Her antiquity, her poverty, the disorganization of her community, and the systematic neglect that she had suffered were all of a higher order of magnitude than anything we had experienced before. One did not have to be a particularly keen observer to sense the special plight of Lincoln.

Located in an industrial slum known as Mott Haven to demographers but called nothing in particular by its denizens, the main building of the hospital dates from 1894. It has been renovated, augmented, painted, partitioned, and renovated again down through the years but it remains indisputably turn-of-the-century in feeling and function. Next to the main hospital, dwarfing it somewhat, is the Nurses' Residence. Constructed in 1927 to house the no longer operative Lincoln School for Nurses, the now ramshackle structure rises ten stories to a colonnaded roof that invokes a grandiosity, a magnificence that clashes absurdly with present-day life in the South Bronx. The "hospital complex" is completed by two dumpy former factory buildings which house the Mental Health Services and some administrative offices.

On one side the hospital buildings are bounded by a decaying but picturesque row of ancient brownstones. The remainder of the hospital is rimmed by the ugliest elements of modern city life—the eight-lane Bruckner Expressway, a large and noisy bread factory, and the terminal garage for the Yellow Cab Company. America's airlines add the final insult to Lincoln's ecology: the South Bronx lies in the center of the approach pattern to La Guardia Airport. All day every day at three-minute intervals the noise of a low-flying jet shatters the quiet of the wards.

Lincoln, I remember thinking, was void of amenities—physically, financially and, most important, medically. No one spent time at Lincoln for optional diagnostic exams of nonspecific aches and pains. No one sojourned at the hospital to recover from a little anxiety or a bad family spat, as they might at other hospitals in other communities. Lincoln was a front-line triage station. To be admitted to share in the hospital's Spartan facilities a patient had to be extremely ill. In my first week at Lincoln I was walking past the Emergency Room on the ground floor when the swinging doors burst open and a black man came staggering out into the corridors and fell to his knees. A medical intern, a friend of mine, followed close on his heels and helped the man to his feet. "Leave me alone, Mister. I can do it myself. I've done it before." The man had a severe tremor and could barely support himself on his emaciated legs. He had blood caked on the corners of his mouth. He wove down the hall grasping a hand rail when his tremor would permit, heading resolutely toward the exit. The intern followed helplessly. The man paused in a waiting area by the door and dropped himself onto a bench.

I stood in the corridor and watched the incident. The intern stopped by me and shrugged. "He's an old wino who's sober. There's nothing we can do. My problem is to decide if he can get home in a taxi or if he needs to go in an ambulance." He followed his patient to the door.

Perhaps the strongest sense of the impoverishment of the hospital that we all experienced on arrival was the on-call rooms. All hospitals that employ a house staff provide quarters for the interns and residents to use on the nights they spend in the hospital. In my experience on-call rooms are of about the same style and comfort as patients' rooms. Fancy hospitals have plush rooms for the house staff and poorer hospitals offer simple rooms. This axiom held in spades for Lincoln; we all shared small rectangular rooms on the fifth and sixth floor of the Nurses' Residence. The rooms had two beds, makeshift desks, a single light bulb in the ceiling, and peeling paint. I was lucky to have an antique brass fan in the cubicle I shared with Marty. It ran on direct current—the only electricity available in the room. Electric razors were out of the question. Men and women took turns in the bathroom. The showers were ancient spigots that dumped a single jet of water onto the cracked tile and plaster of the bathroom floor. The shower room had no curtains, no heater, and no fans. Its walls and ceiling sported mammoth cavities where the plaster had long since vanished. The rooms on one side of the building opened over the expanse of the Bruckner Expressway where the din of the traffic was oppressive at all times of the day and night. The rooms on the other side faced the ambulance ramp where sirens fractured the night at regular intervals. Cockroaches were everywhere.

The poverty of the on-call rooms was only a purgatory for us. We accepted it gamely, often being too tired to notice when we finally reached our beds. But the wretchedness of the hospital itself was a different question altogether. Patients using the Emergency Room, the clinics, and the wards came not by choice but by necessity. They risked their lives, not just a night's sleep, at Lincoln. And to them it could not have looked very different than it did to us—a battered, dirty, old, overused, understaffed institution. A kind of subway station of a hospital. They told us frequently and usually apologetically that people in the South Bronx called Lincoln the Butcher Shop.

Who could object? A patient arriving at the hospital with a pain or a fever not considered an emergency could easily spend three hours waiting to be seen. The adult Emergency Room was always a disaster area treating a steady stream of gunshot wounds, stabbings, auto accidents, and heart attacks in almost no space. High above the doors of the central holding area someone had hung a large, second-rate, landscape oil painting in a baroque wooden frame. It stared inappropriately down over the pandemonium that often prevailed beneath. The patient with a problem that was not an acute emergency was screened out and sent to "Section K," a 200-foot-long narrow corridor with examination cubicles opening off one side of it. There the "nonemergent" patients would sit on one of two rows of plastic chairs facing one another waiting to be called. The corridor also served as the principal passage to all the other clinics in the hospital. So, the "nonemergent" patient with his pain would sit quietly on a chair, keeping his feet carefully tucked in so that no one would step on them, and wait to be called. It often took the better part of a morning or afternoon.

The Butcher Shop. It was a catchy phrase, a supportable conclusion for folks who needed no medical degree to describe what they saw —beds in the halls, beds in the corridors, excrement backed up in the toilets, graffiti carved in walls, cracking plaster everywhere, a fetid Diarrhea Room on the pediatric ward where cases of diarrhea were treated together because there were no isolation rooms. The *New York*

Daily News and *La Prensa* described the details of heart transplantation. Everyone watched "Marcus Welby M.D." and "Emergency Room" and saw the slick face of modern American medicine. But when sickness called in the South Bronx, it was Lincoln—Lincoln, a hospital that looked more like an armory or an abandoned factory than a center for the healing arts.

Lincoln's problems were more than skin deep. As I came to know the hospital and how it functioned, it became harder to dispute the Butcher Shop conclusion. A decade after Intensive Care Units and Cardiac Care Units had been accepted as a key to salvaging critically ill patients, Lincoln had but a single eight-bed unit to treat all severely sick patients. Surgeons, internists, and pediatricians were forced to scrap among themselves to gain admission for their sickest charges. The equipment for the special care of cardiac patients lay crated in the hospital basement for lack of space and administrative will to set up a Cardiac Care Unit. We admitted children to the unit only reluctantly because of the absence in Intensive Care Unit of nurses trained in the care of children. Two floors below, space existed for a Pediatric Intensive Care Unit, but it lacked equipment and nurses. The administration turned it into a locker room. The Recovery Room, a standard hospital facility for the immediate post-operative care of surgical patients, was open only during the day shift because of budgetary constraints. Patients operated on late in the day or emergency cases done during the night were generally wedged into the all-purpose Intensive Care Unit, diluting the quality of care for everyone. Clearly and significantly, no one who had any responsibility for running the hospital had any intention of ever being hospitalized at Lincoln themselves because no one with any knowledge of what is available medically today could possibly be satisfied with the intensive care capability at Lincoln for themselves or their families.

A scandal that both the community and the hospital authorities could agree on was the discovery that the newly painted walls of the pediatric wards contained a level of lead that was illegal for retail paint. It exceeded all acceptable criteria for interior paint. Lead poisoning is an endemic disease in the South Bronx. Children contract it by eating chipping plaster and paint impregnated with lead from the time when there were no ordinances to regulate the level of lead in paint. We regularly admitted children to treat their lead poisoning and to remove them from the environment where the lead was available. As it turned out, it existed in abundance in the pediatric ward.

More than most hospitals, the style and personality of Lincoln were defined by its patients. Missing from Lincoln were the cavernous lobbies and hallways with the busts of important benefactors and men of science. Absent also were the plush waiting rooms with comfortable chairs and racks of magazines. There were no potted plants, no swift elevators, no coffee shops, no gardens, no solariums, nothing in fact but hard plastic chairs placed in the narrow corridors of the ancient building—and the patients. Lincoln's patients and their problems *were* the hospital. They came to Lincoln for one reason—the alleviation of pain. They had no ulterior motives, no hidden agendas. They came in desperation. More often than not they brought with them a complex of problems far more burdensome than those of the patient arriving at the usual general hospital. They were the people of the slum. They were not the simple peasants of some poor but integrated rural society. They were not the proud tribesmen of an emerging nation. They were the denizens of the South Bronx, escapees from the American South or American Puerto Rico, drawn lemming-like to the city, to New York. Unable to speak the language, jobless, the target of layaway plans, pimps, and hustlers of every sort, they moved into the South Bronx, where there was the highest rate of heroin addiction in the world. They lived there in squalor—a special American urban squalor, tempered and, to some, justified by occasional color TVs, big cars, washing machines, stereos, and the like. And when they got sick, they came to Lincoln.

Many patients, of course, came to Lincoln seeking help for straightforward medical problems. Many, though, came looking for aid with troubles discussed little or not at all in standard medical texts—drug addiction, lead poisoning, "hyperactivity," street violence, alcoholism, vandalism, drop-out children, joblessness, and so forth. The medical staff at Lincoln and the Collective in particular knew they were not dealing with the average population and, given the paucity of their training and the poverty of the resources, tried to work with the problems they faced. Like the intern debating whether the patient was so sick he had to go home by ambulance, we all faced many ludicrous and infuriating situations. These scenes told much about Lincoln and its patients but they also revealed much about the system of medical care and social welfare in our "advanced" nation.

Josefita Flores was a five-year-old patient of mine, crippled in the first year of life by tuberculous meningitis. Retarded to the point where she could only smile and cry, gnarled so that she could only roll or creep, she lived with her mother and four brothers and sisters on the fifth floor of a walk-up tenement near Lincoln. Their block was an urban atrocity, their building a wreck, and their apartment crumbling around them. Besides her family there were two things in the world that really mattered to Josefita's well-being. The first was her hospital bed. A year or two before she had finally outgrown her baby crib and her mother had placed her on a regular bed. Since she could roll but had neither the judgment nor the coordination to control her movements, she often fell to the floor, punishing herself pointlessly. Mrs. Flores finally took the mattress off the bed and placed it on the floor. This proved no solution since Josefita became a constant target for rats and roaches and, on one occasion, she rolled off the mattress against a radiator and burned herself badly. Finally the Welfare Department obtained a hospital bed and delivered it to the apartment. It turned out to be an adult-sized hospital bed rather than the oversized crib she should have received. The slats were wide-spaced and Josefita regularly caught her head, her arms, or her legs between them. Mrs. Flores was happy with the improvement, however, and refused to renegotiate the bed for fear of losing it.

The other significant item in Josefita's life was her wheelchair. Like the hospital bed it was a relatively new piece of equipment but, unlike the hospital bed, it was entirely appropriate to Josefita's needs. The wheelchair provided her with an alternative to endless hours of wallowing in her urine-soaked sheets and staring at the walls and ceiling. She could be strapped upright in the wheelchair and pushed to any part of the house to observe the family or look out the window. More than this, it offered her the potential of visiting the outside world. Transporting Josefita was no longer as easy as it had been when she was an infant. She had become a thirty-five-pound dead weight and it was out of the question for her mother to carry her any great distance. Therefore, the wheelchair provided her with transportation outside the apartment. Her visits to see me at the hospital, for instance, were always in the wheelchair. Any trips made anywhere for any reason were dependent on the wheelchair.

But Josefita lived on the fifth floor. Transporting her, to say nothing of the wheelchair, down and up four flights of stairs was an impossibility for Mrs. Flores alone. As a result, Josefita had become a virtual captive of her dying apartment. Knowing the situation, I tried to help Mrs. Flores with her application to the city for public housing. Public housing means housing projects that are built and maintained by the city. Ugly and often dangerous, housing projects are still highly desirable to many families living in even worse situations and the number of applicants is always greatly in excess of the number of available apartments. For the Floreses a housing project apartment would have offered the special advantage of an elevator. Mrs. Flores's application had been pending for several years without any sign of success. In an effort to get the application moving I called the supervisor of the Applications Section of the City Department of Housing. She did not know the Flores family at all but promised to look into the case. To my surprise, she called me back of her own volition about a week later. She explained that she had reviewed the entire situation and in view of the circumstances, she had determined that it should be given a higher priority. Therefore, the case was to be upgraded to a category known as "extreme medical emergency." I was delighted with this and asked her what the chances were that the Floreses would get new housing in the near future. She paused, and then said: "A family of six as an *extreme medical emergency* . . . there is no chance they will get housing in the near future or, in fact, in the foreseeable future." We talked a bit more. She suggested that if I had any political pull or knew anyone who did that I could attempt that, but through standard housing channels the picture was bleak. It annoyed me that she wasn't more upset, but the housing dole was her job and I suppose if it bothered her she would have quit long before she became supervisor. As far as I know Josefita Flores still lives in her acrid, oversized bed, victim of an eradicable disease, a prisoner of her fifth-floor apartment.

If the case of Josefita Flores was a study in the failure of the social service system, the case of Magdalena Perez was an example of needless parsimony in the face of pain. A gigantic thirteen-year-old suffering from a rare, disfiguring, ultimately fatal illness called Marble Bone Disease, Magdalena lived in perpetual pain. Her adolescent frame was forced to support a 180-pound body topped by a grotesquely overgrown head. The disease had caused the bones of her skull to enlarge uncontrollably. In addition to rendering her face horrible to look at, the affliction slowly closed the orifices in the skull through which the nerves of vision and hearing passed. The result was progressive blindness and deafness. Trailing bravely through the hospital, led by her petite mother, she came to see me at regular intervals. She was always an object of fear and curiosity for the other children in Pediatric Clinic who had less spectacular problems.

I had little to offer Magdalena. The disease process was relentless and not amenable to any curative treatment. But I hoped to do something about the pain. Her feet hurt her constantly. Small and hopelessly flat, they were never made to serve such a large distorted body. Specially built orthopedic shoes offered at least an even chance of accommodating her weight better and reducing her daily ration of discomfort. I wrote the City Department of Welfare, the family's source of support, and suggested that the most important and humane thing that we could do for Magdalena from a medical standpoint was to spend $35 or $40 for a pair of shoes. I outlined her medical situation in some detail and urged them to approve the shoes. I received a prompt response from a functionary in the Welfare Department stating that the Welfare Law did not allow them to make such grants and that I should make "private arrangements" to obtain the shoes. He thanked me sincerely for my interest.

For Josefita Flores and Magdalena Perez, for their families, and for thousands of others who lived in the South Bronx, Lincoln stood as a symbol of the system. Despite an occasional positive interchange with a helpful clerk, a thoughtful nurse, or a conscientious doctor, the building, the staffing, the attitudes and, most important, the system in and around the hospital bespoke Butcher Shop. Whatever Mrs. Flores and Mrs. Perez thought of me as their pediatrician, the fact remained that I could not help them. Ultimately, neither they nor I could dent the system. The medical care that society offered them and for which Lincoln was the symbol was grudging, stingy, generally impersonal, and degrading in many ways.

Lincoln has not always been the Butcher Shop. For almost a century after its inception it had been a charity institution controlled by a philanthropic Board of Managers. It was high charity—white, female, and wealthy—and it thrived and expanded.

The Society for the Relief of Worthy, Aged, Indigent Colored Persons met for the first time in 1839. They resolved to found a home for runaway and freed slaves who were arriving in New York in increasing numbers and whose "indigence and unobstrusive sufferings" they had witnessed. The home, located on the Lower West Side of Manhattan, took in its first charges in 1842 and grew steadily through the middle years of the nineteenth century. In 1860 the institution moved to newly constructed buildings at First Avenue and 60th Street. The custodial character of the care gave way slowly to a growing medical concern so that in 1882 the name of the expanded institution was changed officially to The Colored Home and Hospital "in view of the thoroughly organized medical department." The 1890s saw age and demand overtake the buildings on the East Side of Manhattan. There is suggestion in some accounts that Board members and realtors alike felt that a "colored" institution should be more appropriately located on the outskirts of the city on less valuable land. In any case, the Board purchased a lot in the Bronx at 141st Street and Southern Boulevard and built a new hospital. In 1898 The Colored Home and Hospital made its final move to its present location. Commentators of the time described a long and touching column of elderly black men and women moving slowly up Fifth Avenue and across the Harlem River carrying all their possessions with them. The commissioner of the State Board of Charities, speaking at the dedication ceremonies, reflected his rather frugal view of the project: "I have no hesitation in saying that there is no superior class of buildings in this State *devoted to charitable purpose.* What I especially commend is the *simplicity of the structure showing proper economy* of building, convenience of all parts, which suggest precision of administration and improved sanitary arrangement in all the details of the entire group." (Italics added.)

Despite the fanfare, the move to the Bronx soon proved an error in terms of the basic mandate of the institution. No blacks lived in the semi-rural South Bronx. Transportation was marginal and the new location was literally miles from Manhattan's black population. The "economical" wards of the new building remained largely vacant from the time of occupancy. Bound as they were to the new structure, the Board initiated a series of changes that, in time, would spell the total diversion of the original intent of the institution. These innovations would turn the charitable home for colored people into a city hospital.

First, application was made to the City of New York Department of Charities for the support of patients. This was awarded at the rate of sixty cents a day for medical patients and eighty cents a day for surgical patients. Second, a horse and buggy were acquired and offered for use of the local community as an ambulance service. Third, and most significant, the sixty-year-old institution changed its name to the Lincoln Hospital and Home thereby offering its services to whites while maintaining an echo of its Abolitionist origins. "There is no change of management," wrote the Secretary of the Board.

The same love exists toward the colored race, but it has grown broader and more inclusive. There is room for every applicant and better possibilities for help in time of need. Come one come all is still our invitation, but if there be empty beds we need not because of color refuse hospitality to any of God's creatures.

The Home Wards, which were residential or chronic care wards, remained exclusively black but the Hospital Wards gradually grew to reflect the racial make-up of the predominantly white South Bronx neighborhood.

In line with these developments, the medical routine of the hospital began to change. Admitting and visiting privileges were extended to local physicians. A house officership program was started and expanded steadily over the years. The hospital's first chapel was converted into a "modern dispensary" which eventually developed into an Emergency Room and an Out-patient Department.

Coincident with the move to the Bronx was the opening of the Training School for Nurses, the first school for black nurses in the United States. The initial class of twelve entered in 1898 and graduated in 1900. Students had to have a letter from a clergyman testifying to good moral character and approval from a physician "certifying sound health and unimpaired faculties." The young women worked twelve-hour days receiving seven dollars a month "for dress, textbooks, and other personal expenses . . . and it is nowise intended as wages, it being considered that the education given is full equivalent for the services rendered."

Early fears that black nurses would not be able to find employment proved false. Lincoln graduates easily gained jobs in all aspects of the developing field of nursing. The school grew and flourished, expanding to a three-year curriculum and receiving recognition from the State Board of Regents in 1905. In time most of the nursing positions in the hospital as well as the Training School came to be occupied by Lincoln alumnae. Other graduates became leaders in nursing and nursing education around the country.

In spite of the many developments in and around the hospital, charity remained the financial blood of the institution. Authority and responsibility rested in the hands of the well-organized, energetic Board of Managers, all of whom were wealthy white women. They raised funds, gave donations, served on committees, and visited wards frequently. The Phyllis Pavilion, for instance, for the care of patients with tuberculosis was given by "A Friend" in memory of a black servant named Phyllis. "What a tribute to faithful, loving service is this building," wrote the secretary of the Board in 1899, "with its bright sunny wards, its cheerful outlook, its especially careful and scientific treatment of that fell disease to which the colored race so readily succumb."

But the many rapid changes occurring at Lincoln in the first decades of the new century were to prove ruinous to the hospital's financial and administrative core. Functioning in most respects as a municipal hospital, receiving all comers, covering an ambulance district, providing emergency services, Lincoln's Board of Managers experienced growing difficulty in making ends meet. Moreover, the mission of charity at Lincoln became increasingly confused. While preference was given black patients, the hospital had become a community hospital for an area with little black population. Then, too, the Abolitionist sentiments on which the hospital had been founded had eroded considerably by the start of the new century and the final reports of the Board of Managers relate severe problems with fund raising. In 1925 the Board of Managers of the Lincoln Hospital and Home sold the institution to the City of New York Department of Public Welfare to be run thereafter as the Lincoln Hospital. "The work begun for the Old and Indigent Colored People is not as necessary as it was in 1839," stated Mrs. Henry Stimpson, the last President of the Board. The managers of Lincoln, however, agreed to carry on their work at the Training School for Nurses, investing what resources they had in it. "It is seen that a more helpful work for the colored race," wrote Mrs. Stimpson, "can now be carried on by a more specific work for the young colored women in training them for a larger life of opportunity and usefulness."

For eighty years Lincoln was a straightforward charity hospital providing what appears to have been an efficient and dedicated medical service. It seems unlikely that its patients of those years would have thought Lincoln a Butcher Shop, since the hospital offered a reasonable and well-run rendition of medical care as it was available in the late nineteenth and early twentieth centuries. Moreover, the plant was up-to-date and the medical staff comparable to that to be found in other parts of the city—features not present at Lincoln in later years. Lincoln's managers from the 1840s to 1925 were stereotypes of similar boards that developed and directed institutions for the poor throughout this period. Devoted to the hospital, paternalistic and affluent, their style was both the strength and the ultimate weakness of the enterprise. These women and their industrialist husbands were sufficiently strong and adequately rich to provide good service—for a time. But ultimately private charity proved unequal to the task of running a hospital. At that point they were forced to abandon the effort and turn the hospital over to an ill-prepared city government.

The City of New York, in essence, continued Lincoln as a charity hospital (initially, in fact, it was run by the city's Department of Charities) but the charity rapidly became part of the welfare system, which meant maintaining some of the worst aspects of the charitable heritage—paternalism, absentee control, superciliousness—and eliminating some of the best—personal involvement and individual commitment. Like private charity, welfare was a dole, but a dole largely stripped of the human touch. Nowhere in either system was it suggested that the individual patient or the community around the hospital had any particular rights as far as medical care was concerned. Such medical service as could be provided with the charity dollar or with the Department of Charities (subsequently the Department of Hospitals) budget would be meted out at Lincoln but the recipients of that care were not to have any particular say as to the amount or use of those funds. The transfer of Lincoln from private hands to city sponsorship was, in fact, achieved with little or no reference to patients or community.

To some degree welfare represents a principled and idealistic way of helping the less fortunate while at the same time it is a mechanism for keeping paupers and incurables off the streets. Welfare institutions protect both the well-being and the conscience of the more affluent classes. City and county hospitals are no exception to these maxims. For example, Bellevue, New York's oldest hospital, was founded expressly as an asylum for the quarantine of the diseased poor and infested travelers who might pass their afflictions on to the rest of the city if they were not removed from the streets.

Quarantine and protection are not very sound principles on which to found a complete system of medical care, particularly from the point of view of the objects of the system, the poor. But that is where the story of welfare medicine begins, and it was these principles that led to the system of finance and management to which Lincoln fell subject in 1925. Significantly, the welfare system, like the charity system, did not define or recognize medical care as the right of the recipient. Both saw the provision of care as a duty of a sort. Lincoln's old managers might have called it their "mission," while the city saw it, grudgingly, as their statutory responsibility. That difference in attitude would go a long way toward explaining the erosion and decay of medical care that were to take place at Lincoln over the ensuing forty years.

The advent of city control meant new lines of authority for the hospital. Lincoln came under the directorship of a Medical Superintendent. He was responsible to the Commissioner of Hospitals who, in turn, reported to the mayor and the Board of Estimate from whom he derived his funds. The assumed role of the community—to the extent there was one—was, as with all city agencies, through the traditional political apparatus—city functionaries, elections, and patronage. Theoretically the average patient with interest in the hospital or a complaint about it could approach his local City Councilman who, in turn, would address the issue to the appropriate person in the Department of Hospitals. The department would then make a decision or a recommendation and send the message back to Lincoln. In theory at least, the patient would have influenced the direction of the hospital. In fact, this system was far too circuitous and impersonal to afford any real consumer input to the hospital. At base, no mechanism existed under the welfare system of hospital management to overcome the distance between the patient and the system. Such accountability as a critic—patient or otherwise—might have found in the Board of Managers disappeared with the advent of the city.

The years following the city takeover were, according to all reports, ones of slow medical decline. Lincoln continued its tradition of medical education, graduating a group of resident physicians each spring who went forth to practice private medicine as in years gone by. The ties between the hospital and private physicians, however, slowly weakened as the patients became increasingly non-paying wards of the city rather than private patients of the local doctors.

During the Second World War the number of available interns and residents as well as senior physicians fell sharply. Services were curtailed and the quality of care deteriorated. A rapid turnover in city administrators during this period permitted further slippage in health care and the hospital program. But the war years and the period following them spelled far more important changes for Lincoln. For the first time since the hospital opened half a century earlier it began to serve black patients in significant numbers. The black migration from the American South that characterized this epoch brought thousands of black families to the South Bronx. They mingled un-easily with the variety of ethnic minorities that comprised the pre-dominant population of the area and, as has been the case in every American city, the whites soon left. Young people with families de-parted first, leaving the elderly and, often, the sick. (Even today there is an occasional impoverished octogenarian immigrant from Central Europe living in a dilapidated room in the neighborhood who receives his medical care at Lincoln.) By the mid-fifties the South Bronx was a black ghetto.

The black hegemony in the area was short-lived. Hard on the heels of the black migration came a Puerto Rican immigration of equal magnitude. Economic conditions in Puerto Rico, combined with the advent of cheap air transportation from the Caribbean, attracted Puerto Ricans to New York City in rapidly increasing numbers during the fifties. The South Bronx, already a decayed neighborhood, be-came home by default to the influx of Spanish-speaking people from predominantly rural backgrounds. By the mid-sixties Puerto Ricans outnumbered blacks in the area and today there are roughly two Puerto Ricans to every black in the South Bronx.

It was during the fifties that Lincoln reached its nadir as an institu-tion. In every regard it became a welfare hospital. Its philosophy, clientele, financial base, and style were welfare at its inevitable worst. The building itself was hopelessly outdated, the last major renovation having been made in 1934. Funds had been earmarked by the city for the construction of a new Lincoln in the late forties. Those monies, however, never arrived in the South Bronx, a community with little weight in New York's power politics. Instead the city chose to build the 1400-bed Bronx Municipal Hospital Center (comprised of Jacobi and Van Etten Hospitals) on 63 acres of parkland in the white, quasi-suburban Northeast Bronx. In a final insult to the South Bronx, Dr. Marcus Kogol, the Commissioner of Hospitals who was most responsible for developing the new city hospital complex, resigned to become the first dean of the new Albert Einstein College of Medicine being constructed across the street from the Bronx Municipal Hospital Center.

The medical staff at Lincoln declined steadily in both numbers and abilities. Private practitioners abandoned the South Bronx at a rapid rate during the post-war years. Ties between the shrinking private medical community and the hospital staff became increasingly remote while, at the same time, fully trained physicians showed little interest in staffing the decaying, impoverished nonacademic medical center for blacks and Puerto Ricans. Interns and residents, the backbone of most welfare hospitals, shared these sentiments. Moreover, the growing emphasis on scientific medicine drove house staff physicians toward university affiliated programs and away from community service hospitals such as Lincoln. The result, again mirrored in most city and community hospitals around the nation, was the importation of increasingly large numbers of foreign medical graduates to staff the wards and the clinics. These physicians would endure a year or two at Lincoln in the hope of moving up the hierarchy of American hospitals. The Lincoln experience also offered them an opportunity to familiarize themselves with American medicine and to improve their English. To their credit they served (and to a very great extent still serve) where Americans would not. This contribution cannot be denied. But in general their abilities, their level of communication with their patients, and their long-term commitment to the South Bronx was poor.

By any standards Lincoln was run terribly during this period. A frank report on Lincoln by the State of New York Department of Social Welfare in 1958 has captured and preserved the flavor of mid-century welfare medicine. The investigators observed in part:

Bathing and toilet facilities throughout the main building are inadequate. There is one bathroom for each ward. (Census ranging from 30 to 48.) In these patient bathrooms, there are three sinks, three toilets, two tubs and one shower. However, the tubs are discolored, water is running and in some areas only one tub could be used. It is doubtful that any of the patients use these facilities. None of the showers can be used. These toilet rooms are also used as a personnel locker room. Lockers are lined up along the walls and personnel must dress and undress in this room. These rooms have still another function as they also serve as the patients' lounge. Theoretically patients are not permitted to smoke on the wards. (However, several bed patients were found smoking during rounds.) Therefore, if a patient wishes to smoke he must do so in the bathroom. As a result this area is quite congested as up-patients spend a great deal of time sitting in wheelchairs, on window ledges and other places chatting and smoking. Patients have no other recreational areas or places to go. The bathtub and shower areas are also used for storage areas for old and broken equipment or equipment that is no longer in use. *This diversified use of a bathroom is most unusual and most undesirable.* The doors to all toilet rooms should be vented to help circulation of air. Male and female toilets are not indicated on outside of doors. (Italics added.)

And further on, with either thoughtless naïveté or purposeful understatement, they reported:

A tremendous amount of adhesive tape is used to repair equipment. Handles are made for drawers out of adhesive tape; rags are stuffed in windows and held in place by adhesive; doors are held together by adhesive; furniture is repaired by adhesive. *This is an expensive use of adhesive tape and certainly adds to the unattractiveness of the units.* (Italics added.)

The fifties also saw the demise of the Lincoln School for Nurses. Over the years a larger and larger share of the budget of the school had been assumed by the city. The structure of the school remained that of an independent institution run by Lincoln's old Board of Managers, affiliated with the city hospital. But by the early fifties the city was paying $1,424 per pupil each year to keep the school afloat. An effort to close the school in 1950 was narrowly averted in New York City Council with the argument that the hospital itself could be run more cheaply because the school provided sufficient free labor to allow Lincoln to function with fewer nurses than it might otherwise. In 1956, in order to meet the rising costs of education, the Board of the school requested a budget increase of $450 per student because, the Board reported, the original endowment of the school was exhausted and increased city support was required to keep it functioning. This time the Department of Hospitals did not support the school in the City Council debate. Instead they claimed that Lincoln was a segregated school and therefore had no business being open anyway. In the history of the School for Nurses to that time there had been only one white student, a policy never challenged previously by the Department of Hospitals. The director of the school from its founding until 1953 had always been a white woman, until 1953 when Mrs. Ivy Tinkler, a Lincoln graduate, became the first black director. Born of racism, endowed for the education of blacks, heritor of the bitter aspects of American racism, it stands as one of the cruel ironies of Lincoln's history that its School for Nurses, one of the few places a black woman could find nursing training for half a century, was closed with the excuse that segregated education was not acceptable. The City Council refused the request for funds and the school was phased out in 1960.

It was during the age of welfare medicine at Lincoln that its patients began to call it the Butcher Shop. Lincoln clearly had become a terrible hospital. The very permanence of the term Butcher Shop, bequeathed by Eastern Europeans to blacks who, in turn, lent it to the newly arrived Puerto Ricans, suggests a stoicism, a hopelessness, an acceptance that Lincoln was the best that America would give them. By the late fifties even the crassest city administrator had to admit that Lincoln was a shambles and that something had to be done about it. The something, as it developed in the next decade, was the "affiliation program."

Lincoln was not the only Butcher Shop in New York in the fifties. Lincoln's poverty of management, its antiquity, the decay of housing, and the distintegration of institutions in its neighborhood were, perhaps, worse than the circumstances surrounding other city hospitals in New York, but the basic deterioration of welfare hospitals, the flight of doctors from the inner city, and the drift of interns and residents to university hospitals were occurring throughout the city. In 1959 Mayor Robert Wagner chartered the Heyman Commission (named for its chairman, David Heyman, an influential medical philanthropist, and directed by Dr. Ray Trussell of Columbia School of Public Health) to investigate the situation in New York's municipal hospitals and present the city with some suggestions for a cure. The Commission had little difficulty in ascertaining and describing the horrendous conditions that existed in most city hospitals. The tough part of their job was recommending to the city what to do about what they found. Their answer was to "reestablish" the city hospitals as teaching institutions. The only likely source of medical manpower to staff the hospitals, they reasoned, was interns and residents. In order to attract well-trained, American-educated house staff, medical schools would have to run the programs. Therefore, New York's medical schools and voluntary hospitals would have to be invited into the municipal system as affiliates of the city— hence the affiliation program.

The city bought the affiliation idea and made its author, Dr. Trussell, Commissioner of Hospitals. He set about developing contracts to staff each city hospital with professionals from New York's private medical centers. The contracts granted the medical center a sum of money to supply medical staff for the municipal facility. This meant that the private institution was given the job of hiring house staff, attending physicians and such support personnel as were deemed necessary for the city hospital—a large responsibility by any measure. In time six of New York's seven medical schools and eight of its private voluntary hospitals bought into the system. Initially the contracts were financially attractive, since there was little monitoring of the city money. As a spate of studies in the late sixties showed, the private institutions tended to use the funds to meet their own priorities rather than those of the hospital or community.

For the city system as a whole, the affiliation scheme meant a great deal more than a simple staffing tactic. It certified, once and for all, the premise that municipal hospitals would be manned by house officers. Lincoln was no different in this regard from any of the other city hospitals but this fact is highly significant in examining the subsequent developments at Lincoln. In essence the affiliations simply meant that it was no longer possible to lure mature physicians into the system as anything but teachers and that the bulk of patient care would have to fall, by default, to the only remaining category of graduate physician—the house officer. This had tremendously important implications for the style and quality of care in New York's city hospitals.

Lincoln, as can be readily imagined, was not a hotly sought-after hospital for the purposes of affiliation. Albert Einstein was the only medical school in the Bronx and while it already held the affiliation with its neighbor, Jacobi, Lincoln also fell to its dominion. The new program began in steps. The Einstein Department of Pediatrics with Dr. Einhorn in attendance began working at Lincoln in 1958 several years before the affiliation program became policy. The Einstein Department of Medicine, on the other hand, did not get around to doing anything at Lincoln until the affiliation was a number of years old. Theirs was the last section to affiliate, the link being established in 1965.

What, in fact, did the affiliation achieve for the hospital? On the positive side, it is fair to say that at first it did accomplish its stated goal of attracting more and better trained house staff to Lincoln. It did this partly by the agreed-on formula of hiring teaching physicians of medical school caliber for Lincoln and partly by simply including the ghetto hospital in the rotations of interns and residents at Jacobi-Einstein. Some Lincoln departments (pediatrics, for example) continued to hire their house staff to work solely at Lincoln while others were staffed entirely by rotators from Jacobi. The dedication and quality of the physicians thus obtained was variable, some working because it was the only job they could get, and others serving grudgingly, biding their time until they returned to Jacobi. Nevertheless, the overall numbers and the general credentials of the post-affiliation medical staff were unquestionably superior to those of the pre-affiliation hospital.

A second area in which the affiliation succeeded at Lincoln was in establishing a more flexible, albeit redundant, administration. For a variety of reasons the traditional city administration at the hospital could do little in the way of innovation. They were locked into a series of fiscal, bureaucratic, and character restraints that precluded responsiveness to medical or technical developments. Einstein set up an administration of its own to oversee the funds and personnel that it deployed at Lincoln. Ward clerks, unit managers, translators, additional lab technicians, physician's assistants, and even nurses were hired under the Einstein administration, allowing the hospital to keep pace with some of the developments in medicine. The system, to be sure, was Byzantine—the city hiring the college to make the innovations in the city's own hospitals which it could not make itself—but changes did take place. The Einstein-employed workers, of course, had a separate pay scale, different supervisors, and a union of their own. These factors, neglected by the authors of the affiliation, became irksome and destructive in time. At the outset, however, it appeared that the city had bought an efficient, aggressive, private agent to effect some overdue changes in the antiquated Lincoln Hospital.

In sum, the affiliation achieved a degree of modernization and improvement in the medical esprit and abilities of the hospital staff. As one veteran Lincoln orderly put it, "You should have seen the difference the college made when they started here. Before we had dirty old beds in the aisles, in the halls, and everywhere. Now we have beds in the aisles but they're *new* beds."

A number of things can be said against the affiliation scheme. First and foremost is a flaw in the affiliation concept itself. There was indeed a tragic stalemate in the city hospitals in the 1950s. The remedy tendered in the affiliation concept, however, was predicated on the acceptance of two systems and, likely, two levels of medical care in New York—public and private. Good medicine, the definition went, was private medicine. The practitioners who had left city hospitals knew that. The house officers who sought their medical educations in private institutions knew that. The public, who avoided city hospitals if they could, knew that. The possibility to challenge that notion and reverse that trend existed at the time of the affiliation decision. There were eighteen city hospitals with close to one-third of all New York's patient beds, an expanding population eager for services and a tremendous capacity for education in the health sciences. The sad state of affairs in the city hospitals could have been rectified by establishing an independent system of public medicine that would have served as a model for other cities and counties with public hospitals. Rather than relinquishing control of their hospitals to private forces the city might have tightened control, hiring such medical educators, efficiency experts, and technicians as they needed. To improve staffing they could have increased salaries, provided scholarship incentives, developed paramedic and nurse practitioner programs. Instead of handing over authority to outside interests who had no real stake in the city system, they could have incorporated community residents and agencies into the directorship of the various hospitals and into the Department of Hospitals itself. This would have provided the feedback and criticism essential to a responsive system. They should have built new hospitals where new hospitals were needed.

Why did the city hospitals not go this route? Money is not the answer. The reforms proposed surely would have cost money. But nothing could have been as expensive as the affiliations with the city paying essentially unpoliced monies into private hands with generous allowances for overhead to pay salaries largely set by the private institutions. It would have required an incredibly ambitious city scheme to have outpriced the affiliations. The city did not select an independent route of reform because that would have challenged the power and the prerogative of the private medical institutions in the city. Besides, no one in the city government or the private institutions believed in the possibility of an independent system of public medicine. No city in the United States had one. In fact, no city in the United States supported nearly the number of hospitals that New York did. Therefore, if the New York system was in trouble, the logic went, the best answer was to look back to private medicine for help. To move in the other direction would be foolhardy. That argument prevailed. So it was that the city Department of Hospitals called on the private sector of medicine in the person of the medical schools and the voluntary hospitals to enter the system and, for a handsome wage, run it piecemeal in accordance with its own private and individual standards.

A second major shortcoming particular to the Lincoln affiliation was the specific relationship of Lincoln to the Einstein-affiliated hospitals. The affiliation program throughout New York has been criticized for the tendency to relegate the affiliated hospital to second-class status by comparison with the private hospital in the match. These problems have, indeed, existed between Einstein College Hospital and its affiliated neighbor, Jacobi. But Lincoln stands yet another step removed from the primary locus of power within the Einstein empire. Jacobi shares a campus with Einstein while Lincoln is located ten miles across the Bronx. Jacobi has 1,200 beds and was designed as a medical school hospital whereas Lincoln can hold only 350 patients and was built in the last century as a home for freed slaves. Jacobi serves a large and disparate community that has no common identity and little self-awareness. The hospital has experienced no push for community control. Lincoln, by contrast, is a community hospital in every sense. Its patients, who live on every side of the hospital, have increasingly demanded a role in the running of the hospital. All of these factors diminish the appeal of Lincoln within Einstein's multiple affiliation arrangements. She is the poorest sister of poor sisters. The differential in service could be seen daily in virtually every aspect of hospital life—the level of medical school input, the skill and accountability of administration, the vigor of recruitment efforts, the laboratory facilities available, the condition of house staff quarters, and so on.

It is hard, perhaps, to appreciate the shortcomings of the affiliation "solution" to the problems of city hospitals without having worked under the system. Certainly I had no sense of the situation prior to leaving Chicago. New York with its eighteen city hospitals appeared to be a city of medical progressiveness. The involvement of New York's medical schools in the city's hospitals seemed to me an admirable act of social commitment and community responsibility. After four years working in New York's city hospitals and several more to think it over, I do not retreat from the premise that medical school involvement in city medicine is good and important for the level of care in public hospitals and for the medical and social training of the students. Medical schools did not create the two classes of care that city versus private medicine mandates. But they do to some degree benefit from it and help perpetuate it. It is essential for analysts and reformers of America's medical system to understand that. And so long as the public/private division exists it is crucial that institutions of learning and young medical workers remain involved in the public system so as to observe it, to improve it where possible, and one day to change it.

Every institution needs administrators. I was not so much of an anarchist as to believe that enterprises as complicated as hospitals can run themselves without the presence of key individuals charged with planning and coordinating the myriad activities that take place within the institution. The administrative staff of a hospital runs an intricate business that requires food, linen, surgeons, diapers, fresh blood, telephone operators, birth control pills, and straitjackets (to mention only a few items) in order to operate smoothly. They simultaneously direct a hotel, a restaurant, a laundry, often an ambulance service, frequently an institute for higher education in the medical sciences, as well as a medical and surgical service. Their mission includes long-range planning, budget and finance, settlement of grievances, union negotiation, and the like. The medical and nursing staff are, of course, responsible for their immediate areas but the hospital—the well-being of the hospital—is the charge of the administration.

If a business fails, one reasonably asks, "And what of the management? Where did they go wrong?" If a hospital is a Butcher Shop it seems fair to question the administration. Who are they? What are they like? What is their commitment to the hospital?

Lincoln never lacked administrators. Since the affiliation, the hospital has supported two complete sets of administrators, one hired by the city and the other by the College of Medicine. The twin authorities comfortably overlapped and reduplicated themselves in many areas. More important, their existence promoted large voids where each administration conveniently claimed the other had responsibility. The result was paralysis in many trouble spots that badly needed action. The two teams were unmistakably different in temperament and style although their purposes dovetailed well enough so that they lived together amiably.

The Collective was anxious to learn more about the financial problems of the hospital. We approached the city administration asking that someone knowledgeable be assigned to lecture us on the fiscal situation at Lincoln. We were told that the perfect person was Dr. Samuel Blake, the assistant administrator in charge of patient billing. Our ambitious plans for a formal noon-hour presentation with the entire department present received a setback when it was learned that Dr. Blake worked the night shift and was willing to meet with us only between eight and nine in the morning. So we gave up our grand scheme and a small group of us went to meet Dr. Blake in his office early one morning.

Dr. Blake might have been created by Charles Dickens. Graduate some forty years ago of a now defunct medical school, he was at the tail end of an undistinguished medical career. He had practiced medicine briefly during the Depression and, finding it difficult and unremunerative, had turned to medical administration. He had not seen a patient in thirty years. After brief efforts at a number of administrative posts he had found his way into the New York City hospital system. After twenty years of labor, mostly at Lincoln, he had risen to the post of Assistant Administrator for Billing and Patient Accounts. Blake worked only at night. That way, he explained to us, he avoided the many problems of dealing with people and he could get much more accomplished. The evening shift (four to twelve) was not tranquil enough for him. He had to work "the Graveyard," midnight to eight A.M. He looked a creature of the night, small and sallow with a wizened face punctuated by protruding eyes. He greeted us wearing a green eyeshade and drab suit pants supported by suspenders. His office was absolutely barren of decoration. A single, bald light bulb in the ceiling lit the room. He had no desk—only a series of tables stacked high with patient charts.

He approached warily. Why had we come? What did we want to know? And why? We explained to him that we were interested in learning about the finances of the hospital. Did the patients pay? Did Medicare and Medicaid pay? How self-sufficient was the hospital and how much money did the city have to supply? We wanted to know these things, we told him honestly, because we were interested in Lincoln and thought they were subjects that the house staff should know about.

He circled slowly. Lincoln had changed. People had changed. Billing was ever so much more complicated than before when you simply gave a patient a bill. Life, in fact, was more complicated than before. With about that much general information (if it could be called information) he launched into a furious diatribe about "them." "They are liars and cheats," he insisted. "It wasn't so bad in the days before the 'giveaways' [Welfare, Medicaid, and Medicare] because people couldn't cheat. Now it's insufferable. My job is to hold the line against the cheats, against the conniving, malingering handout hustlers. They're everywhere." He processed the many requests the hospital received for medical information pertaining to disability, veterans' pensions and Workman's Compensation. He bragged at length about how few people swindled the taxpayers and the insurance companies under his regime. He simply declared them in good health and their money stopped coming or never came at all. It was his greatest achievement and he was proud of it.

We sparred a little with Dr. Blake, suggesting that everybody wasn't a cheat. He ignored us and rambled on. We asked him again about the hospital finances. He stuck strictly to his personal opinions about patients. "What difference do budgets make when the patients are out to get you? They'd take the chairs out of the waiting area if they weren't nailed down. Somebody has to take a stand." Promptly at nine o'clock he rose and put his suit jacket on. He had had a long night, he told us, and he had to go. We left amused but staggered that this grizzled old man worked through the small hours of every morning blocking as many benefits as possible for Lincoln patients while we labored during the day trying to support and strengthen the same people and families. The elderly doctor rarely had an audience and he seemed to have enjoyed talking to us.

All the administrators were not as earnest as Dr. Blake. Mr. Ira Goldman had been a lawyer. Now he was Lincoln's Assistant Administrator for Administration. Mostly he was the hospital's Notary Public. I met him by accumulating parking tickets. The word was that he could help you get the fines reduced, but his skills were vastly overrated. He lived in Queens where he dabbled in real estate and commuted to the Bronx, which he considered an inferior borough. He had done it for years. Affable, portly, and white-haired, he suffered an apparent addiction for white and two-toned shoes. He seemed to wear a different pair every day. Invariably they blended terribly with his baggy suits and drab ties. Goldman had been at Lincoln longer than Blake and knew everybody. His administrative duties seemed to center on his twice-daily "rounds"—tours of the hospital where he strutted, gossiped, and mostly flirted with the nurses or receptionist in every clinic and on every floor. He often carried a dirty cartoon or an obscene joke scribbled on a piece of paper in his pocket. He loved showing his profanity to mockingly outraged women at every stop on his trip. Rarely called to meetings (even by the administration) he was always to be found in his office except when he was "rounding." When I stopped in his office I never found him doing any work. He always sat at his empty desk and chatted with his secretary, who shared his small office and was a gossip herself. He would notarize a document quickly and return his instruments and the quarter (the fee) to a box in the top drawer of his desk. Then he was ready to chat. Leaving quickly was virtually impossible.

The college administrators were quite different. Dr. Alan Zimmerman was in his late thirties, balding, stout, and apparently efficient. He swept everywhere in his white coat, mimicking a clinician. He never saw patients, though, and was rarely seen in the hospital, preferring his administrative suite across the street or his office at the college hospital. He handled the details of the affiliation contract between Einstein and Lincoln. Though trained in internal medicine, he tired of patients quickly, preferring the palace intrigue and money shuffling of academic administration. He lived in Westchester and did not like the commute, which was made somewhat more tolerable by his Mercedes sports car. The car stood out in the parking lot at Lincoln and was a favorite target of the omnipresent battery- and tire-snatchers. He left Lincoln after a year and a half to become vice president of a firm manufacturing medical instruments.

Einstein learned something during his tenure. It had been a period of community protest and unrest. They decided it would be better, or at least simpler, to have a Puerto Rican in Dr. Zimmerman's position. So they selected Dr. Jaime Valpariso, an affable, rotund, elderly psychiatrist who had worked briefly with the Lincoln Mental Health Service prior to his appointment as Affiliation Administrator. It apparently mattered little that Dr. Valpariso had never done any administrative work before. His appointment, like many at Lincoln, was not made to solve problems but to avoid them. With a Puerto Rican heading the Einstein presence at Lincoln, the medical school felt more comfortable.

Aside from the ineffectiveness ordained and promoted by redundant administrations, the major import of the affiliation arrangement at Lincoln was the transfer of a tremendous quantity of authority away from the city into the hands of Albert Einstein College of Medicine. In my four years at Jacobi and Lincoln (both in "the Einstein complex") I knew of no intentionally malevolent use of Einstein's power over Lincoln. Nonetheless, Einstein did not do well by Lincoln. The interest of the medical school was simply different from and sometimes contrary to the interest of the South Bronx community. Einstein ran Lincoln in keeping with its own interests. The decisions made, the bias exercised, did not always serve Lincoln well and did, in part, allow Butcher Shop medicine to continue in the South Bronx. Let me illustrate.

Head trauma is epidemic in Lincoln's neighborhood. Auto injuries (mostly to kids playing in the street), violence, and violent crime involving the head, and "sky divers" (children falling out of tenement windows or off tenement rooftops) make skull injuries common in Lincoln's Emergency Room. Lincoln perhaps more than any hospital in the city needed an expert head trauma team. But the treatment of injuries of the skull and brain is extremely expensive, requiring the presence of neurologists and neurosurgeons, massive X-ray equipment for diagnostic tests, and an efficient Operating Room and Intensive Care Unit. Since Lincoln lacked most of these services and since they all exist within the "Einstein complex," the medical school decided that head trauma should not be treated at Lincoln. Patients suffering head injury (or any other neurological problem) were to be shipped uptown by ambulance, a risky voyage at best. We once tried to save a child dying quickly from a blood clot on the brain by drilling her skull with the only drill available—a dentist's drill. We failed. The head trauma situation at Lincoln was resolved by Einstein with a logic satisfactory to itself, but not consistent with the needs of the South Bronx.

The city administrators as well as the decision makers at the College of Medicine consistently showed an inordinate belief in gadgetry. Of course, machinery comes easier than people and for the five or ten thousand dollars that it costs to employ a human being for a year you can buy some pretty fancy and durable pieces of metal and plastic. Moreover, machines don't have politics, tenure, unions, or race. The pediatric wards, for instance, sported two exquisite bed scales designed for metabolic research work. The scales were built into the bed in such a way that a patient could be weighed to a thousandth of a kilogram without ever removing him from the bed. These machines resided on a ward that not infrequently saw shifts with no nurses, where the training of nurses barely dealt with the concept of weight loss in diarrhea let alone the workings of a metabolic balance, and where house officers were, reasonably enough, satisfied by weight in ounces and not thousandths of a kilogram. And the scales became hopelessly inaccurate due to their frequent rough use by interns weighing themselves when the beds were empty.

In the Out-patient Department one day an entire bank of seats was removed from the waiting room area in order to store ten crated microfilm readers that suddenly appeared. A tenuous affair at best, Lincoln's Record Room suffered chronic understaffing and inadequate space that made the retrieval of information chancy in general. No hospital records were then on microfilm. Rather than dealing with the space and manpower problems of the Record Room, some well-budgeted front-office type had seen fit to renovate the medical record system with microfilm readers. So he sent ten of them to a clinic area that had fourteen examining rooms. If there had been records on microfilm to be read and if there were some sensible way to divide ten readers into fourteen rooms there might have been some use for the machines, if they would have fit into the small examining rooms—which they did not.

Beyond the problem of gadgetry, though, and beyond the questions of decision making, the basic query that remains to be asked of Lincoln after ten years of affiliation with Einstein is: What is the level of care like as a result? Has the system been sufficiently renovated so that reasonable, contemporary medicine is practiced? It is easy to cite isolated events at any hospital to suggest good or bad medical care. Anecdotes alone are not a good yardstick of medical practice. But the tale of a ten-year-old Puerto Rican girl I helped care for at Lincoln goes beyond simple anecdote, beyond the indictment of a single person or department, to suggest the real systemic neglect that has continued under the affiliation program. The child was admitted to the hospital on a Saturday afternoon suffering severe crush injuries of the chest as a result of an automobile accident. The surgeons took her to the Operating Room immediately where a prompt, creditable job was done removing bone fragments and blood clots from her collapsed lung. Following the three-hour operative procedure she went to the all-purpose Intensive Care Unit (on Saturday, the Recovery Room was closed). Because of the damage to the lung and her depressed state of consciousness following the accident and the operation, she required assistance with breathing. To this end we attached her to an artificial respirator, an air pump coupled through a series of valves to a small tube inserted in her windpipe by way of her mouth. The pump itself was driven by compressed oxygen from a bedside tank. The respirator supplied extra oxygen when the child breathed but, additionally, had a timer that tripped the machine to breathe for the child if she failed to inspire in four to five seconds.

For the twenty-four hours following the surgery the child's condition remained serious but stable. On Sunday night, however, an alert went out over the hospital page system indicating a cardiac arrest in the Intensive Care Unit. When we arrived we discovered a nurse attempting to resuscitate the child, who had stopped breathing. We quickly disconnected the respirator and with external heart massage and manual artificial respiration, using a hand pump, we got her heart started again. We then reconstructed what had happened. The nurse reported noting that the respirator was silent and that the child was receiving no air. The heart stopped beating and she called the emergency alert. This was a strange situation, since the respirator was set on automatic and would continue to pump air at five-second intervals even if the child had died. A quick check revealed the only possible circumstance that could explain the silent respirator—the oxygen tank that drove the respirator was entirely empty. The child died soon thereafter.

An explanation for this situation was poor nursing, but the background to this death involves much more than just poor nursing. Granted, decent nursing would have noted the low oxygen tank in advance and ordered a fresh one. There was, however, an Oxygen Therapy Department in the hospital whose job it was to supply and restock oxygen tanks. Where were they? An intensive care nurse should be familiar with every aspect of artificial respirators since many of their patients use them and since she is often alone without physicians in the unit. How was it that this nurse could not diagnose the obvious problem of a silent respirator meaning an empty tank? The Anesthesiology Department is responsible for all problems of assisted ventilation and, therefore, should play an active and vital role in the Intensive Care Unit. In point of fact, this nurse had never received a moment of formal instruction from the Department of Anesthesia. The anesthesiologist on call that weekend had played no role in helping the medical and nursing staff care for the child. At a subsequent meeting called to discuss the death of the patient, it was revealed by the acting director that the directorship of the Department of Anesthesia had been vacant for six months (an area of Einstein responsibility); apparently no member of the department was clearly in charge of the Intensive Care Unit; and there appeared to be no program of nursing education on the subject of respirators. Such knowledge as existed in the hospital on the subject of respirators seemed to be entirely random. The final salient fact in the respirator story is that the use of bedside oxygen tanks is an entirely obsolete practice in all hospitals. At Lincoln in the late 1960s a central oxygen facility was installed in a parking lot adjacent to the hospital building and oxygen jacks were installed on the walls of the wards over the patients' beds. Somehow the administration had never seen to it that the central unit was connected with the bedside outlets. The result was the continued use of portable oxygen tanks. The failure of the system at Lincoln on every level allowed this ten-year-old resident of the South Bronx to die.

Has Butcher Shop medicine at Lincoln been replaced with something better? Are the changes in the hospital more than skin deep, more than *new* beds in the halls, more than useless microfilm readers in the clinics? From my experience the answer is no. The affiliation has not triumphed over the Butcher Shop. The affiliation, rather, has been a dodge, a clever step sideways. The basic issues of Lincoln's charity heritage and the failure of public medicine in America have neither been confronted nor overcome by affiliation. To the contrary, the basic problem of charity medicine in the midst of a predominantly private system has been obfuscated by the entrance of the private medical schools into the city system and has made the resolution of the problem less likely and more expensive. The affiliation program has not changed the system; it has simply given it a new custodian.

A senior physician now on the staff of Lincoln relates a story of a recent trip to Africa on vacation. Flying from Dar-es-Salaam to Addis Ababa, she happened to sit next to a well-dressed, middle-aged man. He turned out to be an American living permanently in Saudi Arabia, employed by an oil company. He warmed noticeably when he learned that the physician worked at Lincoln Hospital in the Bronx. The oil executive, it seemed, had been born at Lincoln and brought up in the South Bronx by European immigrant parents. He had only one question about Lincoln. "Tell me," he queried the physician without a trace of embarrassment, "is it still the same old place? Do they call it the Butcher Shop?"

7

Seize the Hospital to Serve the People

When the Collective arrived at Lincoln in July of 1970 to begin work it was not, as many later contended, the beginning of political activity at the hospital. A significant amount of unrest, dissent, and anger had surfaced in and around the hospital in the two or three years prior to 1970. Moreover, the agitation was not the work of a single group but rather spontaneous eruptions brought about by unrelated groups. Militant demands for change at Lincoln preceded the arrival of the Collective by several years.

In July of 1969 a cabal of angry workers in the Lincoln Community Mental Health program took over their service and demanded the ouster of its leaders—two psychiatrists—and a series of reforms making the program more accountable to the community. The immediate result of the uprising was the arrest of twenty-two persons and the firing of sixty-seven more. Eventually, most of the workers were reinstated and the psychiatrists in question were removed. The most important outcome of the "mental health strike" was not the changes in the department but the drawing together of a group of people who were to be instrumental in subsequent events at Lincoln. These individuals were for the most part young, black or Puerto Rican community mental health workers whose political outlook and grievances were varied. Following the mixed outcome of the strike they began to work more intimately with the Black Panther party and the Young Lords organization. This experience developed both their own internal discipline and the breadth with which they defined the problem; that is, they saw the situation at Lincoln not simply as a badly run city hospital but as part of a larger health struggle, part of the way that white, well-to-do bureaucrats dealt with black and Puerto Rican people. They began to talk increasingly of community-worker control of Lincoln and Third World leadership in health actions.

A second, unrelated insurrection took place at Lincoln in April of 1970. At that time the position of Hospital Administrator was vacant, a post always occupied by a white professional appointed by the Commissioner of Hospitals, and a group of community people decided to challenge the tradition. Their candidate was Dr. Antero Lacot, a middle-aged Puerto Rican gynecologist with a master's degree in public health and experience running a community maternity center—hardly a radical choice. The Commissioner of Hospitals refused to support him and the Committee for Lacot swung into action. With the press in heavy attendance, they sat-in in the hospital lobby in a show of determination to get their man appointed. Twenty-two were arrested and carried out to police vans. Significantly, the groups backing Lacot were neither Lords nor Panthers. They were representatives of forces totally different from those activated in the mental health strike. Mostly they were members of Puerto Rican community organizations or political clubs that existed in the orbit of Ramon Velez, a local political boss of considerable power who hoped to extend his influence within the hospital with a director chosen by him. But the demonstrators had real grievances against Lincoln—grievances important enough to make them willing to be arrested for them. And in the end they were successful. The mayor overruled the hospital commissioner and Lincoln had its first Puerto Rican administrator.

During this same period in 1970 plans were afoot for the establishment of a community board for Lincoln. The Department of Hospitals recognized that there was growing unrest concerning the hospital in the increasingly political South Bronx. Part in cunning, part, perhaps, in fear, they moved to appoint their own Community Advisory Board for Lincoln. The Commissioner of Hospitals selected the members of the board and, virtually without exception, chose individuals representing established interests in the South Bronx—established businesses or political factions, churches, poverty programs, and so forth. Few if any of the appointees actually received their medical care at Lincoln. The hospital's staff and workers had no representation on the board. Moreover, the board had no real duties or powers that related to the day-to-day management of the institution. Finances, hiring, medical policy, planning, and grievances all remained in traditional channels, unaffected by the existence of a community board. Meetings of the board were irregular and, generally, ill-attended. Rather than establishing a legitimate tension between the community and the forces that ran the hospital, they served to rubber stamp hospital policy and insulate the Department of Hospitals and Einstein College of Medicine from growing demands for change taking place in various segments of the community.

Both at its inception and later, Lincoln's Community Advisory Board was flawed in many ways. One activist critic called it "too little too soon," implying that a much sounder, more legitimate board could have been established if events had been allowed to generate a grass roots demand for a community board. Yet the formation of the board in early 1970 was another proof that the powers downtown recognized that the community was restive and that they were not going to accept broken-down medical care in the decade to come as they had in the decade past.

Even as the Collective arrived at Lincoln to begin work, community pressure on the hospital was mounting. In June, the month before the Collective arrived, a group calling itself "Think Lincoln" began a concerted action in the hospital. They met with the newly appointed Dr. Lacot and informed him of their intention of setting up patient complaint tables in the lobby of the hospital. Without waiting for a response they went to work. "Think Lincoln's" style was direct action. Comprised of a number of people who had been involved in the mental health strike as well as several black and Puerto Rican activists from the South Bronx community, they saw their task as hospital reform, not by petition to the established authorities—including the Community Advisory Board—but by direct appeal to the patients and the community. The complaint table was intended as a mechanism to stimulate patient awareness and participation in the hospital.

They put their table in the center of the ambulance-emergency room entrance of the hospital where the majority of patients were likely to arrive. Colorfully decorated with bilingual signs and staffed eighteen hours a day, the table was immediately obvious to everyone in the hospital—worker and patient. "Think Lincoln" stocked the table with a variety of leaflets and pamphlets discussing patients' rights, alleged hospital abuses, and community control. The signs invited grievances and reminded patients that the hospital was *their* hospital.

The "Think Lincoln" action was, predictably, the source of immediate tensions in the hospital. Many physicians saw the tables as an act of impertinence and ingratitude. Accustomed as they were to having no feedback from their patients, the action frightened them. Hospital workers were of mixed opinions on the subject. Some were enthusiastic while others reacted defensively. For many patients the complaint tables meant little, but for a few it changed the role of the hospital in their lives. For all patients it was a symbol that some- one was trying to deal with the problems of Lincoln. Complaints were handled directly and promptly. If the complaint was considered rea- sonable, a "Think Lincoln" member would accompany the patient to the clinic or ward in question and discuss the problem with the ap- propriate staff member. Most often this resulted in an explanation or rectification of the problem. Occasionally things did not go smoothly. One noonday a number of patients complained about the three-to- four-hour wait in the Adult Screening Clinic, the notorious Section K. A check revealed that only one doctor was assigned and he was eating a leisurely lunch. A group of four representatives from "Think Lincoln" went to the doctors' dining room (the doctors still had sit- down service in a room of their own) and, in loud voices, demanded volunteer physicians to staff the Screening Clinic. Several doctors responded angrily and a chin-to-chin confrontation resulted which had to be broken up by the hospital Security Police.

Generally, though, the "Think Lincoln" campaign was not disruptive to hospital life. While many physicians and workers took the challenge personally and felt their individual work was being questioned, they could live with the complaint table. Others saw the campaign in perspective and concluded that anything that focused attention on the shortcomings of the hospital would benefit medical care in the long run. These staff members were friendly and supportive to the "Think Lincoln" effort.

The "Think Lincoln" action embarrassed the Community Advisory Board. They could not disagree with the demand for articulation and redress of patient complaints. Even the undertone of community con- trol that pervaded the campaign was in keeping with some vague rhetoric of the Community Advisory Board. But they generally dis- liked the style and the politics of the group carrying out the action. Moreover, the complaint tables entirely upstaged their own com- mittee. To the very considerable degree that the Community Advisory Board was wed to the system as it stood, they found the complaint tables threatening and radical. The result was paralysis. While it would have been hopelessly compromising to condemn the action, the Community Advisory Board did not have the gumption to support it. The result was official silence.

Very much the same political situation trapped the newly appointed administrator. Alleged champion of community rights, he could not condemn the action or call on the hospital police to stop it without risking loss of face. On the other hand, the pressures from the city and the college to stop the "disruptive" activity were considerable. He, too, equivocated, allowing the continuation of the complaint table campaign.

The Collective arrived to begin work on July 1, 1970, in the midst of the "Think Lincoln" action. In some respects it was more than we could have hoped for. In part, we were coming to Lincoln in the hope of joining hands with the community to change and improve the hospital. The community, it seemed, had already made a move. They had articulated their criticisms and they were doing something about them. Moreover, they obviously needed allies within the hospital to legitimize their claims and help sustain their effort. Clearly there was a ready-made political role for the Collective. Yet, in other respects, the timing of the campaign was unfortunate. The month of July is a trying and even dangerous time in any hospital that relies on interns and residents for staffing because it is the traditional turnover month. Everyone has just been graduated to a new level of responsibility and is relatively slow and inexperienced at the new job. Beyond that, in July of 1970 the vast majority of the Pediatric Department at Lincoln was new to the hospital and more or less new to one another. We had barely gotten our feet wet medically or politically when we were called on to start making some hard choices about the use of time and resources. Clearly and enthusiastically our support went to "Think Lincoln" and the complaint table approach. Yet I cannot escape the conclusion that our efforts would have been better coordinated and significantly better received by the rest of the hospital staff had we had a chance to establish ourselves medically and develop our own collective discipline before we were tested politically.

But events moved too quickly. Marty and I were both on duty on the night of the thirteenth of July. Early on the morning of the fourteenth (we would later joke that it was Bastille Day) we were jarred out of our sleep by someone banging on the door of the Nurses' Residence cubicle that we shared. It was barely light. Marty asked who it was and, hearing no response, we both went happily back to sleep. The phone rang at seven to awake Marty who had to relieve the pediatrician on duty in the Emergency Room. "We've been liberated?" I heard Marty say. "What are you talking about?" He hung up and went to the window. "Fitz! Come here and look at this." I got wearily out of bed and went to the window. The ambulance ramp below was jammed with police cars. Police vans and more patrol cars filled the street beyond. Policemen wearing baby-blue riot helmets milled about the hospital grounds below. "Schipior in the Emergency Room told me we'd been liberated by the Young Lords. I thought he was kidding. But something must be happening. The cops aren't here at seven A.M. for checkups."

In a dramatic—some would say melodramatic—early morning move the Young Lords working with "Think Lincoln" had, indeed, occupied the Nurses' Residence. About thirty Lords had taken up positions on the ground floor of the building, barricaded all but one entrance, sealed off windows, and announced plans to "run a hospital to serve the people." The early morning knock at our door had apparently been the uninspired effort of a cadre who had been assigned the task of notifying the doctors that the building had been occupied. Marty and I got dressed and went downstairs quickly. The ground floor was well occupied. It had the air of a spirited street bazaar. The place was barricaded with chairs and tables piled high at every window. The auditorium had been converted into a day care center and an infirmary for screening tests for TB, anemia, and lead poisoning. There were a press area, security checkpoints, strategy sessions, marshals with armbands, and so on. Doctors came and went freely. The Lords announced that the building was open to all hospital employees and encouraged all clerical personnel from the upper floors to staff their offices. Most stayed away. And the police massed outside unsure what to do.

The Collective supported the takeover. The Lords never requested formal backing in advance since to do so would have jeopardized the secrecy surrounding the planned action. In all likelihood, though, they counted on a fair amount of support from the hospital staff. And they got it. The Collective never met to discuss the occupation. There was no time. But Collective members visited the occupied area frequently, helped staff the day care and the health care programs, and let it be known to the press and the police that physicians backed the Lords. I, for one, couldn't stay away. The Nurses' Residence suddenly had the fantastic, intoxicating air of a liberated zone. The press was listening; the city was listening; and the Lords had risen up and were telling the stories of the women and children waiting endlessly in the clinic, the old folks dying for lack of a Cardiac Care Unit, the humiliation of the Emergency Room, the flies, the pain, the degradation. It felt good, it felt right, it felt righteous. It was why we had come to Lincoln.

Life in the hospital itself went on unmolested. But both sides understood the symbolism of the takeover. For the Lords and their backers the occupation stood as a challenge to the city to account for the sloppy, cheap, unresponsive medical care they dispensed. Moreover, they demanded of the city not just the grudging provision of medical services but the initiation of community programs to stamp out clearly curable diseases, such as TB and lead poisoning. They asked that the hospital move into the community to search out problems. Midway through the morning the Young Lords held a well-attended press conference to state their aims. They were simple enough: that Lincoln establish a community preventive medicine program, a free day care center for workers and patients, a free breakfast program for children of the community, and health education classes for workers and patients. Late in the morning an unknown occupier stated the argument more succinctly. He painted a bedsheet in one of the on-call rooms with the words "Seize the Hospital to Serve the People" and hung it out the sixth-floor window where it waved and flapped over the Bruckner Expressway for the rest of the day.

The city understood the challenge. The presence of thirty young Puerto Ricans wearing berets and exchanging power handshakes in an administrative and dormitory building didn't really require the day-long deployment of hundreds of police and dozens of police vehicles. Yet, the city knew that not to respond was to risk exposure, embarrassment and, most of all, the stimulation of public curiosity and imagination. Why wasn't something being done about lead poisoning? Why is the TB rate four times as high in the South Bronx as it is in mid-Manhattan? Those were questions the city was happy not to have the press or the public ask. And finally, the presence of the Lords was a territorial showdown. If the Lords could assert their right to be present as a community group in an institution of their choosing, where couldn't they go? What city function would go unchallenged? What area of malfunction would escape exposure? The city had to respond.

And respond it did. All through the day the city "negotiated" with the Lords. The negotiations consisted of vague promises to set up some kind of day care or do some sort of preventive medicine if only the Lords would (please) get out. The Lords doubted the sincerity or the conviction of the city or the hospital administration and they held their ground. At five P.M. Dr. Lacot called the medical staff to an emergency meeting. A hundred or so of us packed into the hospital's chapel, the largest room in the non-occupied or, depending how one looked at it, non-liberated zone. From the questions and discussion at the meeting the staff was clearly divided with the Collective and many non-Collective interns and residents favoring the takeover and much of the senior staff—the attending staff—appalled at the Lords' action. After answering a few questions, Dr. Lacot announced that he had broken off negotiations with the Lords and he had asked the police to enter the building within the next half hour to "clean it out." In a move that surely caught the neophyte administrator by surprise and with a sense of the dramatic moment, a member of the Collective jumped to his feet; "Well we know which side we're on. Let's get to the Nurses' Residence. Now!" With that, almost half the physicians in the room rose, pushed out the crowded doorways in front of an astonished Dr. Lacot and went to join the Lords in their beleaguered building. As we left, Lacot kept mumbling "Gentlemen, gentlemen. Consider what you are doing. Consider the risks you are taking. Gentlemen, gentlemen . . ."

Once out of the hospital building we started to run. We must have been a strange sight, a long line of trotting doctors dressed in varying shades and combinations of white snaking their way around parked cars and police barriers to reach the main entrance to the Nurses' Residence. I wasn't sure why we were running. We sensed an urgency to be with the occupiers, to share the battle that now seemed assured, to stand up to the police machine that would be turned on any minute. Once we all clamored up the steps and into the building the police closed the ranks, moving in closer to the building, donning their riot helmets, and bringing up arrest vans and mounted patrolmen. A hasty summit was held in the center of the lobby of the disputed building. About seventy of us were there—half Lords and half doctors. We reasoned that the hospital administration and the police would not risk the adverse publicity of busting, and perhaps beating, such a large number of physicians who, after all, were not trespassing in their own hospital. The Lords were not so sure. They argued that they had made their points well and that it would be useless to stay in the building and risk mass arrests and beatings. Undoing the effects of a violent confrontation with the police would take months. Therefore, they pushed for retreat and we concurred.

But the question was how. The police completely surrounded the Nurses' Residence and were massed in front of every entrance. Simply walking out of the building at this point raised the specter of arrests and beatings anyway. We decided that the best bet was for a few people to leave at a time, doctors and Lords together. We did just that.

It was a strange sensation walking shoulder to shoulder with a young Puerto Rican woman I had not known before and who I would never see again through the angry, tight ranks of police. They cursed us repeatedly as we walked stiff-backed. They called her "Spanish Tits."

The plan worked and the building was abandoned without violence although we learned later that three Lords walking to a bus stop several blocks away were stopped by the police, pulled into an alley, and beaten. The police immediately occupied the building and the action was at an end. Life resumed as usual in the Nurses' Residence the following day. For a few weeks the administration lamely staffed a day care center in the auditorium to show their good intentions. But they soon withdrew their support and closed it. For several years strips of tape in X patterns remained on windows on the ground floor of the building—the only lasting evidence of the occupation.

The apparent peace achieved by the eviction did not last long. Toward the end of July a young Puerto Rican woman named Carmen Rodriguez was admitted to the Gynecology Service at Lincoln for an abortion. Mrs. Rodriguez was a resident in a neighborhood drug treatment center. She was no stranger to Lincoln, having been hospitalized on the Medical Service two weeks earlier for diagnosis and treatment of rheumatic heart disease which she suffered. During that hospital stay the internists discovered that she was pregnant. Feeling that pregnancy and especially labor were more than her heart could stand, the doctors recommended an abortion. At the time of her admission to the Gynecology Service, however, the internists were not called in consultation. She was treated as a routine elective abortion. The gynecologist, through sloppiness or disinterest, performed a saline infusion abortion, an extremely questionable procedure in a woman with heart disease. The hazard was the inadvertent passage of saline (salt water) into the circulatory system of the patient. Such an event would tax a normal heart but could—and did—prove fatal to a diseased heart. Carmen Rodriguez died at Lincoln four days after her abortion—a tragedy, inexcusable by any standards.

When Mrs. Rodriguez was admitted to the Intensive Care Unit after her "routine" abortion, members of her drug program became concerned. They called a psychiatric resident from Lincoln who also worked with the program and who knew Mrs. Rodriguez. He visited the ICU, discovered the situation, and made it public. The word spread quickly. Here was graphic evidence of Lincoln medicine—the medicine the Lords had talked about, the medicine that the Collective had quickly come to know. The story passed rapidly around the hospital. Even before Carmen Rodriguez died people were talking about the woman in the Intensive Care Unit who had been "butchered." The press covered the death laconically as "Abortion Death Reported by City."

"Think Lincoln" and the Lords were furious. They circulated flyers describing the circumstances of the death and demanding that the hospital administration and the Department of Gynecology account for the "murder of Carmen Rodriguez." The Collective backed the efforts of the community groups at exposure by helping document the medical details of the death and by circulating the flyers calling for explanation.

At length the administration consented to an open meeting at which they would "explain" the circumstances of Carmen Rodriguez's death. They played to a full house of angry community people who stuffed the well-used chapel. The meeting was unique in the annals of American medicine. Certainly it was one of the most extraordinary events during my tenure at Lincoln. I have never seen nor heard of a situation where a hospital staff has been called on to detail the circumstances of a complicated medical case leading to a death to a lay group and then accept cross-examination. There are countless examples of parental surveillance of teachers and numerous cases of civilian review of police activities but I know of no other instance of community examination of publicly employed physicians. Unfortunately, the events leading to the meeting were inflammatory and the community arrived in anything but a dispassionate mood. Yet the fact of the meeting was an important event. It was a troubled, even tortured example of community control of medical services. At the least, it was a real and significant instance of physicians being called to account by community people. The agenda did not flow easily but the very meeting of the two sides to discuss a medical event stood as a victory for community participation in the hospital.

Part in jest, part in earnest, we called the session the first People's Clinical-Pathological Conference (C.P.C.). Just as in traditional medical school C.P.C.s, where a difficult case resulting in death is presented, discussed, and analyzed, representatives of the Departments of Medicine and Gynecology described the by then familiar case of Carmen Rodriguez. Lamely and defensively a number of senior physicians, including the director of the Department of Obstetrics and Gynecology, attempted to sell the position that Mrs. Rodriguez's death was unfortunate but reasonable and medically acceptable. The community representatives were angry but they were also well coached by various members of the Collective. They were conversant with the medical details of the case and also the medical options. Why had a saline induction abortion been chosen for this woman with obvious heart disease? they asked. Why were her medical records not available to the gynecologist performing the abortion? How could it be, they queried, that the physician who first saw her when her lungs began to fill with salt water due to the failure of her heart did not apparently listen to her heart but, rather, assumed that she had asthma and initiated an inappropriate and harmful treatment?

The answers to these questions were halting, compromised, and clearly unacceptable to the audience. Spokesmen for the Lords and "Think Lincoln" argued that Carmen Rodriguez was killed by the system. They charged neither incompetence nor malice by the doctors performing the abortion but insisted that a decent system with accountability to the patient and continuity of medical coverage would have prevented the senseless death. They called it "systematic murder" —murder committed by a malicious system. Therefore, they demanded not the resignation of the doctor performing the abortion, but the ouster of the director of the Department of Obstetrics and Gynecology. They held him responsible for the overall program. They argued that for his $52,000 a year salary and the rank of full professor at the medical school, the city and its people could do better. Additionally, they called for a worker-community board to be established to review and implement the policies and procedures of the department. Finally, they asked that a humane abortion clinic be established and named after Carmen Rodriguez.

Sensitive to the volatility of the situation, the hospital administration equivocated both during and after the meeting. Neither could they deny the thrust of the charges nor did they have any intention of acceding to demands as basic and challenging as those made by the Lords and "Think Lincoln." Shortly after the meeting, a delegation of community people including several Collective members went to the office of the director of obstetrics to pursue the demand that he withdraw. A long session followed at which the obstetrician vacillated, sounding conciliatory at times and contemptuous at others. At the meeting's end a group of angry people, many of them from "Think Lincoln," followed him to the parking lot and, shaking their fists, told him never to return to Lincoln. He let it be known that he did not intend o return. As a result, the residents in the Department of Obstetrics and Gynecology, all of them on rotation from Jacobi–Einstein discharged as many patients as possible, refused all admissions, and abandoned the hospital. The stated reason for their walkout was support of their director and protest against what they termed "intimida ion." For three days the service ran on a crisis basis while negotiations proceeded with the Ob-Gyn staff. At length they returned with an interim director appointed for the department.

Soon thereafter, the hospital administration, acting in concert with the Health and Hospitals Corporation (the new city agency that supplanted the Department of Hospitals in July of 1970), obtained an injunction against any further political activities in the hospital. Cited in the injunction were the leaders of "Think Lincoln" and the Young Lords as well as "John and Jane Doe"—which meant anybody that the hospital administration chose to include. The injunction was open-ended and was to be enforced by arrest. The police were again present in force on the day that the injunction was served. The activists watched the complaint tables dismantled without recourse. For the moment their campaign was blunted.

While "Think Lincoln" and the Lords carried on their program from the streets with leaflets and rallies, another battlefront took shape. An estimated 10 percent of the young adult population of the South Bronx uses hard drugs. Lincoln offered no program to deal with addiction or any of its medical complications. Overdose, hepatitis, infection, and the like were treated piecemeal in the Emergency Room but no department supported detoxification or education programs. Addicts from a number of drug groups in the community came together around the demand that Lincoln provide some sort of drug program. Characteristically, the administration marked time. While agreeing with the premises of the demand, they refused to commit money or space to the program. The South Bronx Drug Coalition, as the group became known, responded by moving into the sixth floor of the Nurses' Residence. The Collective cooperated by giving the addicts keys to their on-call rooms on the sixth floor. The city wasted little time this go-round. With their predictable mono-response, the police moved in and arrested fifteen of the Coalition members and chased the remainder. When I returned to my on-call room the next day I found an articulate commentary on the protest. Marty's and my few belongings were untouched. My bed was rumpled from use and the sink contained a mound of dry, caked vomit, a testimony to the addict's plight. Following the sixth-floor showdown and continued agitation by the Coalition, the hospital turned the Nurses' Residence auditorium over to the drug program. In time, federal monies were obtained to establish a methadone detoxification program.

If the rapid-fire events of July and August 1970 did not result in victory for the community groups assaulting the hospital, they did serve notice to the city and the medical school that there was an angry community ready to contest conditions at Lincoln. During this same period the Collective arrived at Lincoln and began to function medically and politically. In these months of upheaval the Collective was seen variously as the source of trouble, Communist, "right-on," and the hope of Lincoln. The Collective was none of these.

8

Collectivism

What was the Collective? Who was the Collective? How did it work? These questions were asked often following July 1970 since the Collective rapidly became a visible and controversial entity on the Lincoln landscape.

In the fall of 1969, well before the term "Collective" had been connected with our group, we drew up a recruitment brochure. In it we set forth the medical and political thinking we hoped would attract young physicians to Lincoln. "There are an increasing number of medical students and house officers," we wrote,

who have a socially and politically conscious orientation toward their role in medicine, who are concerned with practicing medicine in such a way as to effect social change. However different our political orientations may be, we share a common sense of the need for political change in effecting real changes in an environment which now generates disease. We have found that students graduating from medical school who have been active in various ways while in school have, in internship and residency, become isolated and unable to act in socially effective ways with respect to their work situations. Thus far all we have been able to do while isolated is to adapt and try to survive individually, defending ourselves against the in-humanities which the system tends to bring out even in the best of us. By concentrating a significant number of people with a socially conscious orientation in one hospital and work situation, we hope to create a critical mass of people which will be able to change rather than merely adapt to that situation.

In preparation for this task, the department will reorganize its own structure, ignoring "professional" and hierarchical considerations to achieve an atmosphere where work will be divided intelligently, not dele-gated arbitrarily—where ideas will be exchanged freely and valued for their validity rather than for their source—and where we will be free to focus our energy, not on any individual role with its rigid duties and privileges, but on a shared commitment to the community.

Beyond this recruitment statement we drafted no manifesto or constitution prior to our arrival at Lincoln. Amid the rapid-fire events of July and August we labored rather to build the Collective. The majority of people who considered themselves Collective members were in the Pediatric Department but neither was the department synonymous with the Collective nor was the Collective all pediatricians. There were house officers in the Departments of Medicine and Psychiatry who considered themselves Collective members. A small number of nurses started work at Lincoln during the period around July 1, 1970, with the intent of participating in the Collective. They were joined by several nurses already on staff in attending Collective meetings.

Early on we recognized that the Pediatric Department was *not* the Collective and confusing the two would be troublesome, if not destructive, to both. Significantly, neither Einhorn and his attending staff nor the ten or twelve foreign medical graduates remaining in the department considered themselves part of the Collective. Yet the tangibility of the Pediatric Department (day and night, seven days a week it was a concrete, identifiable entity) as opposed to the somewhat ethereal nature of the Collective (it existed in clear fashion only during its weekly meeting) invited confusion. Unquestionably some Collective members resented the fact that we did not make departmental policy since, after all, we were the majority of the department. Einhorn, on the other side, seemed to lament the independence and strong-mindedness of his new American house staff. Relations with him did not go well from the beginning of July and the pace of events did nothing to improve the attitudes on either side.

We all arrived at Lincoln with many preconceptions about what the Collective would become. The most romantic and ambitious side of those notions was encouraged by the events of the summer of 1970 since it seemed that the community was in revolt and the hospital was ready for our reforms. We failed from the start, however, to assess accurately one key aspect of the situation; we were all house officers, which meant we started each week with a seventy- to one-hundred-hour commitment to direct patient care. What hours we had left had to be divided among sleep, leisure, and the Collective. That did not leave a great deal of time for the Collective—a fact that was to lead to considerable frustration. Put differently, our expectations about our own political output were pitted from the beginning against the small reservoir of time and energy that remained to us after we completed our medical duties. In consequence, both during periods of political

unrest and political tranquillity at Lincoln, the major tangible manifes-
tation of the Collective was its weekly meetings.

Every Tuesday evening at 5:30 we assembled in the Pediatric
Library on the second floor of the hospital. The meeting rarely began
on time because medical chores were not often done by then. And if
they were, the question of dinner came up since our deliberations
rarely finished before 8 o'clock and occasionally ran as late as 9:30
or 10. Understandably, people stole off to the cafeteria to eat before
the meeting. When protest finally arose about our chronically late
starting time people became more punctual, often bringing their
dinner trays with them—a development the cafeteria workers never
appreciated. Attendance varied between twenty and forty as determined by the political situation, morale in the Collective, and the
busyness of the Pediatric Service. With latecomers perching on tables
or squatting on the floor, we sat in a circle on the library's uncomfortable plastic desk chairs. In summer the ancient air conditioner
in the room's one window wheezed continuously, cooling only the
lucky souls directly in front of it. We left the door ajar in all seasons
so we could hear the page operator. Participants were usually tired
at the beginning of the meeting and exhausted by the end; a dozing
Collective member was not an unusual sight. Smoke invariably filled
the room despite our own No Smoking ordinance. The wall phone
rang regularly, calling people away to medical duties.

A typical meeting in the fall of 1970 went as follows: We turned
to serious discussion at ten minutes to six. Fifteen people started the
meeting, including two who were eating dinner on their laps. The
majority of those assembled were physicians from Pediatrics, but a
medical intern and two residents from Psychiatry were present. Joan
Golden, a black woman in her late twenties, representing the "Think
Lincoln" Committee, sat with a sheaf of papers on her lap. Two
young nurses, one black and one white, one in uniform and one not,
sat together at the side of the room. The chairperson for the evening
(the job was rotated on a voluntary basis) was a pediatric intern
named Bob Stanford. He opened the meeting by asking for agenda
items, a ritual we always adhered to although it rarely produced one
half the subjects we eventually covered. A dozen topics were suggested by the group, some of which were relegated to an "announce-
ment" category. People continued to arrive, with a maximum of thirty
present at about 6:30.

Announcements came first. Marty Stein mentioned that Channel

13 (Educational TV) wanted to do a story on Lincoln and had contacted him. Anyone interested should let him know. Joe Wurst (who, in spite of his last name, had an Irish mother) asked anyone interested in contributing funds to the Irish Republican Army to please contact him. Charlotte Phillips announced that the Black Panther party would hold a convention in Washington, D.C., in December and anyone who wanted to go should contact her. A debate followed as to whether we should send a representative of the Collective and it was decided we shouldn't. A "Worker Meeting" in the Pediatric Emergency Room was announced for the following morning at 8 o'clock and one of the psychiatrists invited everybody to a party at his house the next weekend.

Then we turned to agenda items. Paul Bloom reported for the Finance Committee. Paul had become virtually a one-man committee, with the interest of others flagging and his remaining keen. That was typical of his contributions to the Collective. Any project he undertook he carried through with a quiet earnestness. Small, soft-spoken, and short-haired, he in no way fit the stereotype of the youthful radical. Graduate of Einstein, married, with in-laws in the Bronx, Paul resembled a "home-town boy" in the medical school complex much more than the rest of us. He could easily have stayed at Jacobi for an internship and residency and gone on to a lucrative North Bronx or suburban practice. Instead he chose to put his training on the line and do his internship in an experimental program in a little-known hospital. That, of course, was a decision made by all of us, but for someone of Paul's background it seemed particularly unlikely. And it was a decision made seriously because he was to stay at Lincoln more than five years, finishing his training and becoming an attending and a specialist in school problems.

Paul reported that the Collective had $716 in the bank and that thirteen members were at least one month behind in their pledged payments. He then read the names of the truants amid some head shaking. Two people wrote him checks on the spot while several others promised to pay up promptly. The "Think Lincoln" Committee had asked Paul for $500 to print the next issue of their newspaper, *For the People's Health*. He pointed out that the Collective had previously agreed to support the paper and that he wanted to give them the $500. After a short discussion the group concurred.

The Irishman, Joe Wurst, spoke next for the Draft Committee. He, like most of the interns, faced almost certain military conscription at the end of the year if he didn't seek and obtain some kind of deferment. Joe had signed the Pledge of Non-Participation back in medical school and had no intention of joining the military. He and a number of others in the same situation had formed a group to explore the possibilities of medical draft resistance. They talked of coming to live in the hospital and claiming "medical asylum." They reasoned that the Selective Service would not dare enter a ghetto hospital where they were performing valuable service to make arrests and carry them away. Joe reported only that they had contacted a well-known draft lawyer who would meet with them shortly to discuss their problems. As it developed, Lincoln never had a confrontation with the Selective Service, most people obtaining medical or legal deferments of one sort or another.

To this point the meeting had been serious but it had not been "heavy" by Collective standards. That was not to last long; it never did. Bob Stanford next recognized Karen George to speak about the Nursing Service. Twenty-one, wife of a medical student, graduate of Cornell, and veteran of radical politics, Karen had been involved with the Collective from the beginning. "I'm tired of giving the same report at every Collective meeting we come to. I'm sick of laying down the same crap, but that's where it's at." Karen had worked hard to recruit other nurses to Lincoln with her and had succeeded in persuading two classmates to take Lincoln jobs. Additionally, she had been instrumental in getting several of the young, black staff nurses from the Pediatric Department to attend Collective meetings from time to time. One of them, Pat Long, sat beside her but remained quiet during the discussion. "Being a nurse at Lincoln is oppressive to begin with. Dig it? There's the work load, the understaffing, the conditions, the supervisors. The whole scene, see? But the doctors, the Collective, they're supposed to be liberating, together, helpful, thoughtful, supportive. Well they aren't and that's the most oppressive thing yet."

Stanford interrupted her. "What's your point, Karen?"

"The Collective—more precisely, the men in the Collective—do nothing to support the nurses who are women. They act like interns and residents at any piggish hospital in the city. Nurses are for picking up, mopping up, and cleaning up. That's wrong to begin with and it's damned wrong here where there are so few of us. I've said this before but nothing is different now. Every time a doctor starts an I.V., does a spinal tap, or takes an EKG he leaves the Treatment Room a mess—gloves in the corner, paper on the floor, Betadine spilled on the exam table. *You* know what it looks like. There's no reason that stuff can't be thrown away while you work; or if it can't you can spend a couple of minutes picking up behind yourself when you're done. We're not maids."

"She's right," said one of the interns, who was sloppier than average. "We deserve a lot of criticism for the way we treat the nurses."

"Do you guys ever answer the phone on the ward when it's ringing and ringing? Do you ever change a diaper on rounds when you see a baby covered with shit? No, you leave it for us." She paused. "There ain't no way we're going to recruit nurses to Lincoln with regressive, chauvinist shit like that coming down. No way."

A long, self-critical discussion followed in which most people agreed with Karen's points. The angriest diatribe against "pig doctors," however, came from one of the psychiatrists who didn't use the pediatric ward at all. Someone pointed that out to him, which redoubled his wrath. "A revolutionary doctor is a revolutionary," he concluded. "That's all there is to it. Pediatrics, psychiatry, wherever. It doesn't matter. If a woman has to tell you you're oppressing her you've already missed the goddamned point."

The discussion was interrupted by two black men who strode into the room and sat down on the table next to Stanford. They gave Joan Golden in back of the room a fisted salute. She returned it. Stanford asked them to introduce themselves. The first sported an orange dashiki and a bushy natural. "I'm Robert James from the Black Panther party and this is Brother Irudu." Brother Irudu wore dark sunglasses and a black beret. He said nothing. "Three brothers got busted on 138th Street last night. The pig stopped them, frisked them, beat all three of them bad, and then arrested them for resisting arrest and breaking and entering. The real reason the pig did this thing was 'cause they're members of the party. We need $600 to bail them out and we need it quick 'cause they ain't gettin' any healthier where they're at." People responded slowly. Paul Bloom reminded the group that the Collective had only $216 left in the bank after it met its commitment to "Think Lincoln."

Someone else suggested a special collection. Stanford pointed out that if people who owed money paid up there would be more than enough to cover the bail money. "We figured you doctors wouldn't let us down," said James, "because you can dig what it would be like to be beat up sick and sitting in jail at the same time." Finally, Stanford took a number where James could be reached and promised to call him as soon as the Collective had decided what to do. Fifteen minutes after they had come the two black men left.

Stanford asked Joan Golden what she knew about Robert James, Irudu, and the men who had been arrested. She said she knew that James and Irudu were Panthers but she knew nothing of the arrests. She promised to do some checking and let us know. After some more debate it was decided to give $100 of Collective money plus any voluntary donations toward the bail if the three checked out. If they didn't, the donations would be returned.

"Look, it's getting late," said Stanford, "and we haven't dealt with the heaviest thing on the agenda." It was 8 o'clock. "There's something that nobody's dealing with, something everybody's involved in— and everybody's avoiding." Stanford had a penchant for the dramatic. Tall and articulate, people looked to him as a natural leader. The issues he raised almost always produced heated debate, with discussion running toward the moralistic and the personal. "There's been a lot of shit coming down that no one's talking about. It's too important to let slide. It'll eat us up if we don't and we've got to learn from it." Stanford came to the Collective with what he, in his rhetorical moments, would have called "heavy ruling class credentials." Raised on Long Island, son of wealthy parents, he did his undergraduate work at Dartmouth, where he wrestled on the varsity and rowed stroke for the crew. In medical school at Harvard he became increasingly active in the anti-war movement. His conversion to radical politics was cemented during his senior year with an arrest at a peace demonstration. He considered the episode the ultimate proof of his radical commitment because conviction—his case was still to be tried—could prevent him from getting a medical license. As a Collective member he devoted the same kind of energy to radical politics as he once did to athletics.

"Lay it out, Stan," someone challenged. "Say what you mean."

"We've had a lot a dealings with Einstein over the last month, right?" He was referring to the possibility of Dr. Einhorn resigning or being replaced because of disagreements within Linclon's Pediatric Department. Some Collective members had been asked their opinion by Drs. Fraad and Barnett and several potential replacements had been interviewed. "A lot of real liberal shit has been coming down around this whole thing and I think we have to respond to it." "What do you mean, Stan? Are you talking about Sullivan and Rosenbaum?" Sullivan and Rosenbaum were two pediatric residents who had been chosen by the Collective at the last meeting to meet with Dr. Fraad and discuss Einhorn's replacement. Although most Collective members favored his ouster at that point, the group had purposely not taken a formal stand on the question. Sullivan and Rosenbaum were mandated to explore the situation but told to take no position for the Collective.

"I'm talking about the Collective. We've been dealing with the medical school, with the press, with outside doctors and that's very liberal. I mean really liberal of us." In radical circles the word "liberal" was the antithesis of good politics—or radicalism. Liberalism referred to wishy-washy, ill-conceived or self-serving machinations. Liberal bureaucrats, for instance, were those who preached progressive change but who ran programs that prevented that change from occurring by maintaining the status quo. In the New Left, liberals were hated both because they were seen as a slippery and dishonest obstructive force and because most radicals had once considered themselves liberals. "We're being liberal with ourselves because we haven't asked the workers what they think about Einhorn and the department. We haven't asked the community either. Do we believe in community-worker control or not? And yes, I think Rosenbaum and Sullivan were on a liberal trip going up to Einstein. That's liberal and individualist."

"That wasn't individualist, Stan," countered Wurst. "We chose them to go."

"So who are we to choose. Did they talk with 'Think Lincoln,' did they talk with the Lords before they went? Did they ask the workers all over the hospital what they thought before they tripped up to Einstein in the name of the Collective?"

"Now wait a minute, Stan. You're making a lot of judgments. You weren't even here at the Collective meeting when we talked about it last." Stanford missed many Collective meetings, although his presence was felt when he did attend. "Right or wrong, you could have expressed your opinion. And hell, you could have gone up to Einstein if you'd wanted."

"That's not the point. We should never have gone up there alone. Who are we accountable to anyway? I ask again: do we believe in community-worker control? If we do we shouldn't be doing our doctor trips alone."

Since Stanford, the chairperson, was in the middle of the argument, the meeting was no longer being directed and the discussion wandered around the room. "I don't think talking to the people at Einstein was a good idea but not for your reasons, Stan." The new speaker was Bob Goran, a bright second-year medical resident who had come to Lincoln after two years in a prestigious medical residency at Washington University in St. Louis. During much of that time he had lived in a Weatherman commune. The experience had been a difficult one for him. It did not prove easy to play the dedicated young internist during the day and return to the world of the revolutionary guerrilla at night. Since arriving at Lincoln he had become increasingly concerned with personal rather than political revolution. "Our job is to be accountable to ourselves. We can't go around organizing the community and the workers when we don't know each other. We really don't know who we are. I think we ought to spend our time talking about us and if we get done with that then we can talk about Einhorn or the community or whatever. I mean the vibes in here are just terrible. Politics begins at home and that's here for us."

A debate continued for a long time with several people backing Stanford and arguing that *our* opinion about the Pediatric Department didn't matter; that our job was to get the information out to the workers and the community. Action was up to them. Others countered, pointing out the impracticality of that; Stanford's plan, they held, was ideologically pure but would lead to paralysis and inaction. They, in turn, were called opportunist by Stanford's supporters. Joan Golden was asked what "Think Lincoln's" position was on Collective action. She responded that "Think Lincoln" stood for community-worker control (which we well knew) but that the Collective had to decide for itself what actions it would or would not take. The debate eventually ended with a compromise decision that the Collective would respond if events forced our hand but that we would not actively negotiate with Einstein. It was agreed that the topic would be put on the agenda for review at the following week's meeting. No one was really satisfied with our resolve but that was not unusual in such discussions.

It was now ten minutes to nine and only a handful of people indicated they could stay longer; so the meeting was adjourned. There were three agenda items left undiscussed.

It is not easy to characterize the Collective in terms of personalities. All of us had medical or nursing degrees and most of us shared a belief in radical, community-oriented politics. Beyond that, background, motivation and day-to-day practice varied considerably.

Many old friends from SHO days joined our ranks. Henry Kahn (of the "great psychedelic bus" debate) came to Lincoln in 1970 as a pediatric resident even though he had completed an internal medicine internship and first-year residency in Boston. The notion of the Collective excited him and he was willing to start over as a pediatrician to be part of it. Jim Waller (of the "Save Waller's Beard" battle) started as an intern that first year as well. Still sporting his neat goatee, he had graduated from the University of Chicago and stayed on to do two years of graduate work in pathology. He finally decided to complete his clinical training and chose Lincoln, bringing with him far more political and scientific experience than an average intern.

In spite of Collective maxims, however, many people came to Lincoln in 1970 and later for highly personal and individualistic reasons. While some aspects of their political commitment and medical practice helped build and support the Collective, others did not and led, in some cases, to strange and destructive confrontations. At one point a member of the Collective got into an altercation with a black hospital security guard about the intern's failure to wear a hospital identification card. The argument ended in a fist fight and an administrative grievance against the house officer that hardly promoted Collective solidarity with hospital workers. Another example was that of John Jones, an intern in 1970 who had already done a rotating internship at another hospital in New York. He eagerly joined the Collective and happily undertook the repetition of the internship year in pediatrics. From the outset Jones proved a loner in the midst of the Collective. Medically, while other interns were busily reviewing treatment plans with the residents and attendings on their teams, he was devising and implementing treatments on his own. These therapeutic regimens were often inaccurate and occasionally dangerous. Criticism did little to dampen his individualistic zeal. Politically he was unpredictable. Well read in leftist writings, he knew a great deal about the history and the medical system in the People's Republic of China. Yet his behavior with hospital workers was often offensive and puzzling. One morning I received a call from an irate nurse in the newborn nursery where Jones was working that month. Too angry to talk on the phone, she bade me come to the nursery immediately. When I arrived she showed me a pair of well-used socks draped over the lip of a wash basin. "He changes in the nursery," she explained, referring to Jones. "Not only does he change but he airs his clothes too." When I asked Jones about it he replied that he often did change his socks and his shirt in the nursery in the morning. He also brushed his teeth in the same sink. I told him that I thought that was unnecessary, unclean, and absolutely guaranteed to get the staid nursery nurses angry at him and all the "new doctors." That, I pointed out, was a trouble we didn't need with so much else going on in the hospital. In complete seriousness he responded that the nurses (black, L.P.N.s with incomes only slightly above the poverty level) were bourgeois and therefore deserving of contempt. The aides and orderlies in the nursery, he argued, were the proletariat and they didn't mind his activities. He added that in all struggles he was on the side of the proletariat.

For six months he remained an enigmatic member of the Collective, apparently very devoted, always on the radical side of issues, but frequently involved in individualistic episodes such as that in the nursery. At the end of that time he abruptly resigned, stating that he felt there were more important political struggles going on elsewhere that he had to join. His plan to leave was generally met with hostility since his withdrawal meant that other members of the department would have to give up elective or vacation time to cover his slot. Jones seemed oblivious to the bad feeling, spending many days at the hospital after the time of his resignation visiting with friends and attending meetings. Eventually, he left Lincoln and New York with the intent of practicing medicine and politics elsewhere. The Collective, on balance, was stronger without him, but the individualism and arrogance he represented continued to be a problem for the group. In time we became more aware of these tendencies within our numbers and began to focus on them in Collective discussions. Nonetheless, individualism in the midst of collectivism remained an ironic and troublesome issue for the Collective.

Early on we hoped the Collective would become the focus for other forces of change within the community and the hospital. We fantasized that Collective meetings would include nurses fed up with conditions, hospital workers discouraged with the disinterest of their unions in patient care, and angry community residents ready to move on the hospital. Except for a few nurses and an occasional white-collar hospital worker who were allied with the Collective by bonds of race, class, and education, this was not to happen. The Collective and, particularly, its meetings were stigmatized much more than we ever realized. We were, I think, earnest and reasonable representatives of what we were—white, American, predominantly male physicians from comfortable backgrounds with twenty or so years of formal school behind us. Our meetings reflected our background and our bias. They were rambling, contentious, and ambitious of agenda but weak on resolution. The result was that community representatives, hospital workers, and even nurses who came to the meetings tended to be bored and to feel excluded. In time we worked out something of a solution to the problem. Although individuals were never excluded, groups with common interests sent representatives to Collective meetings from time to time to discuss topics of importance to them. We then recognized more clearly what we were—an organization of radical physicians on the staff of Lincoln who were committed to community involvement in the hospital.

The questions of salary sharing and communal living that had been raised at the very first Collective meeting continued to be discussed. They always proved difficult topics because they potentially affected the home life of every person. Income and living conditions were put-up or shut-up issues which made everybody a little uncomfortable. At length, the group voted to let every individual decide what he or she could afford and put it into a Collective account on a monthly basis. Some felt we were being far too soft on ourselves by not setting a tithe and holding everybody to it. Nonetheless, $500 or $600 a month was raised in this fashion and disbursed regularly in support of the Panthers and the Lords, used as bail money for local activists who were jailed, spent to send Collective members to meetings judged relevant by the Collective, and so forth. Although the question of the tithe continued to come up for discussion, the funds we did raise were an important and tangible evidence of collectivism.

Communal living was handled outside of the formal Collective. Early on it was decided that the Collective could not arbitrate living situations. Neither were we small enough nor were we tightly knit enough to take up the questions of everyone's family needs. The idea of communal living intrigued many of us because it seemed appropriate to the lives of people who worked as closely and shared as ardent a politics as we did. Yet the many other considerations of family life prevented many of us from getting involved in communal living. Over the period of two years following July 1970, several groups of people from the Collective did live communally. Some found the experience satisfying while others did not; but in all cases the arrangements took place outside of the Collective and were not part of the Collective agenda.

If salary sharing and, to a lesser degree, communal living were recurrent topics at Collective meetings during the first months, there were countless other subjects that came and went almost before we could talk about them. These, of course, were the many issues raised by the presence of "Think Lincoln" and the actions of the Lords. Unavoidably, we often spent time discussing events that had already occurred and what we could do to follow them up or what we should do if they happened again. Generally the group supported the "Think Lincoln" actions although we sometimes found it hard to respond quickly to their requests for support, which often developed from moment to moment.

We recognized that there was little we could do about this because, in fact, we were reacting to actions initiated by other groups rather than planning actions of our own in response to what we saw at Lincoln. We decided that we should develop our own programs and strategies based on our own experiences at Lincoln. After only a month or two we were well versed in the medical shortcomings of the hospital. One of the most obvious and one that affected both the patients and ourselves in our daily work was the lack of nursing in the hospital. Chronic understaffing of the wards had been the rule at Lincoln for as long as anyone could remember. It was not infrequent, for instance, to have a single practical nurse assigned to cover two forty-bed wards with the assistance of several aides. The problem compounded itself; understaffing promoted understaffing. A new nurse at the hospital would in short order find herself so burdened that she would immediately think about work opportunities elsewhere. The wards were dirty, clean linen was often hard to come by, the neighborhood was tough, and walking from the subway stop to the hospital entrance at night could be dangerous. The hospital system provided neither housing nor transportation for nurses. We documented and protested the situation in a variety of ways, generally meeting with indifference or hostility from the nursing and hospital administration. We recruited some nurses, offered to participate in further recruitment, volunteered to teach in-service training courses, and the like. Our efforts did little to dispel the juggernaut of problems that locked the hospital into its inadequate level of service. We became increasingly convinced that if solutions were to be found there needed to be an infusion of funds, commitment, and energy from the hospital system as a whole. To employ and retain more nurses the system would have to recruit harder, provide housing and transportation, offer incentive and differential pay for tough hospitals (like Lincoln) and for difficult shifts, and generally show a more aggressive posture toward nursing problems.

As of July 1, 1970, the old city Department of Hospitals had been replaced by a sleek, new, semiautonomous Health and Hospitals Corporation. The premise of the corporation was that it could bring savvy to bear on the problems of city hospitals in a way that the Department of Hospitals could not. Atop the corporation was one of New York City's highest paid public officials. At $60,000 a year, Dr. Joseph English made some $10,000 more than the mayor. Late of the Peace Corps and the OEO, Dr. English arrived with good credentials in administrative medicine but with little experience in community or city hospitals. The advent of the corporation generally went without notice on the front lines of patient care in the city hospitals. Perhaps some changes did take place on an administrative level concerning the billing systems and the automation of accounting processes. But the institution of a "firm business hand" made little difference on the wards and in the clinics.

The Collective was instinctively suspicious of the corporation from the start. Cybernetics and big salaries struck us as the wrong direction to move in to solve the city's hospital problems. Moreover, our blunted efforts to counter the nursing debacle seemed to confirm our sense of the corporation's disinterest in the real issues of day-to-day life in the hospital. After much discussion we decided that a contribution we could make would be to call the attention of the city to some of the excesses, inconsistencies, and inactivity of the corporation. With more instinct and reflex than careful analysis, we called on an old and effective friend—confrontation. Using a battle plan that included a detailed floor plan of the offices, entrances, and exits from the Health and Hospital Corporation suite, we plotted an unannounced, face-to-face meeting with Dr. English. We divided our forces so that there would be adequate coverage of the hospital as well as a sizable delegation for the protest visit. With much effort we dictated all our old charts and wrote progress notes on the charts of every patient under our care so it could not be said that medical care suffered because of our political activities. Finally we tipped the press and departed by subway for our late-afternoon sortie on the president of the corporation. Some thirty of us, including a number of patients and community representatives, arrived on schedule and paused briefly to discuss Dr. English's whereabouts with his surprised secretary. We proceeded without formal invitation to the corporation boardroom where we understood the president was meeting. Several reporters and a camera crew joined our assault. Dr. English looked startled to see us. He mumbled a few quick words to one of his assistants and departed through a back door we didn't have on our maps. Several of our group followed him, but he disappeared down a flight of stairs and was gone.

His assistant was left the hapless task of dealing with us and the press. The situation was made worse for him because he happened to be a young physician who had been active in the SHO and had been a good friend of a number of the Lincoln partisans. The meeting consisted of our recitation of the travesties of nursing and medical care at Lincoln and our anger at the corporation for its inaction. Dr. English's lieutenant lamely defended the work of the corporation. The press noted our charges, interviewed a few of us, and took some pictures of angry young doctors in white, which made good copy the next morning. Representatives of the corporation threatened us with arrest and we left. We returned to Lincoln satisfied that we had fought a battle that was legitimately ours. Whether we had won or not was unclear. Neither had the corporation been shamed to death by our assault nor had they dispatched a caravan of supplies and funds north to relieve the beleaguered hospital. We had, though, succeeded in getting a number of our points about Lincoln and medical care through to the public. Moreover, we had added our voice to the growing number that were quarreling with the city over the corporation and its conduct of the public health.

If we were content with our performance at the corporation offices, our department chairman, Dr. Einhorn, was not. Increasingly he found the Collective's actions infuriating and embarrassing. He disagreed with us about almost every event that occurred at the hospital during the long and trying summer of 1970. He considered the complaint tables an impertinence, he could not comprehend the takeover of the Nurses' Residence (which included his office), he opposed community review of the Carmen Rodriguez incident, and he fought to support and retain his colleague, the Director of Obstetrics. The fact that half of his department turned up in the office of the president of the Health and Hospital Corporation was one more infuriating event to him. And with each event the common ground between the department director and the Collective grew smaller. The split between Dr. Einhorn and the Collective (which I think would have occurred eventually even without the events of that first summer) grew because of two significant, separate areas of disagreement. The first was the question of the community and control of the hospital. Einhorn was simply and unalterably opposed to the passage of any power from the hospital to the community. The second subtle but perhaps even more important disagreement developed in the area of style. Einhorn's European, demanding, and paternalistic ways were simply not those of the Collective. Collective members, for instance, were disinclined to call the chief for every moderately tough clinical question they had. They preferred to ask each other, the chief resident or the attending on their team. Einhorn wasn't accustomed to such independence. When he did make rounds on the wards, interns didn't drop everything to follow him—a courtesy to which he had grown accustomed. When he lectured or presented cases from his experience (always a good show), the sessions were often poorly attended—a marked departure from the past. His nursery rounds (his area of specialty) drew scant attention. Einhorn took all this very personally. The Collective was simply not a very academic group of physicians in training. For the most part, the interns and residents hoped to get their work done as efficiently and as well as possible so that they could move on to the many problems generated by the political situation at Lincoln. No one intended to snub Einhorn at the outset; but then no one expected him to be such an overbearing boss. In time people came to resent both his expectations of us and his need for attention. Gradually people did begin to avoid him which, of course, fanned the fires of his resentment.

By early fall, after a mere two months of working together, Einhorn had virtually withdrawn from the service. He gave conferences infrequently, appeared on the wards only rarely, and tended to make rounds with a loyal and preinvited coterie of the remaining foreign residents. Collective members were generally content not to be "oppressed" (a word often used) by Einhorn and continued the chores of patient care without a Chief of Service. By degrees, though, the department entered a crisis. The half dozen attending physicians—loyal to Einhorn, used to his strong hand, and fearing an impending rupture in the department—became restive and began looking for jobs elsewhere. The foreign residents, fiercely devoted to their sponsor, Einhorn, and ill at ease with the Collective and its politics, started to grumble about conditions in general. Matters became worse when a thoughtlessly worded "Think Lincoln" pamphlet on the hospital referred to "foreign mercenary doctors." The entire group of foreign residents in pediatrics threatened to resign. They were badly stung by the notion that they might be considered mercenary and they were angered that any segment of the community might think they were. Particularly embittering was their assumption that the Collective had participated in the wording of the pamphlet. After a great deal of talk, some self-criticism on the part of the Collective and "Think Lincoln," and a round of sincere apologies, the foreign residents decided to stay, but their allegiance to Lincoln was badly eroded while their commitment to Einhorn increased.

As the fall progressed Drs. Barnett and Fraad were presented with a more and more troubling situation. Patient care in the Lincoln Pediatric Department limped along but the teaching program had all but disintegrated. On the one hand, any possibility of Einhorn's backing down or accommodating himself to his new interns and residents seemed remote; while on the other hand, the Collective did not appear likely to accept Einhorn's authoritarian paternalism. Potential remedies reduced themselves to two: either the Collective had to be phased out or Einhorn had to be removed. On a surface level the question became: was it easier to find a single department director or replace an entire house staff at a hospital as decrepit and controversial as Lincoln? While expedience seemed to favor the Collective, allegiance, longevity, and capacity for work favored Einhorn. He had run Lincoln with a skeleton staff before, he could do it again. Moreover, popular or not, he was a member of the medical school faculty and a respected pediatrician. He was one of the fraternity. By contrast, the Collective was new to Einstein, unproven and, to many, suspect for its ideas. It seemed unlikely that Barnett and Fraad would opt for the Collective.

But they did. What tilted their decision in favor of the Collective remains unclear. They certainly never stated what their reasons were, and the rash of charges and countercharges that ultimately followed their decision only served to make original issues more obscure. Perhaps believing that the Collective promised a better future for Lincoln than did Einhorn, idealism motivated them. Others have suggested pure pragmatism forced the decision. The workforce offered by the Collective was too good to pass up and too hard to replace. Finally, some believe that sinister medical school politics dictated the choice: Einhorn was so difficult and so entrenched in his quasi-autonomous sinecure that the medical school welcomed the opportunity to move him out. What the real reasons were for the unlikely decision will probably never be known with certainty. But two items surrounding the choice remain clear. First, the selection of the Collective over Einhorn was not made in such a definitive or unanimous way that it would not be subject to reconsideration under the duress of public exposure and protest. Second, and more important, those making the decision in Einstein's Pediatric Department and the dean's office had no notion of how cunning, tenacious, and bombastic an adversary Arnold Einhorn could and would become.

It took the finding of a qualified replacement who was prepared to take the job to force matters to a showdown. Dr. Helen Rodriguez turned out to be that person. A well-trained, forty-year-old Puerto Rican pediatrician, she had contacted Dr. Einhorn in August of 1970 inquiring about the possibility of a job at Lincoln as an attending physician. Her motives were simple. She had grown up in New York City and returned to Puerto Rico for college, medical school, and her pediatric training. She spent a number of years in academic pediatrics in and around the University of Puerto Rico Medical School, becoming a specialist in the care of the newborn. Coming once again to New York in 1970, she sought a job teaching pediatrics. Lincoln seemed a natural place for her to apply since its patient population was the most heavily Puerto Rican of any hospital in the city. She knew no one in the Collective and learned of the struggles surrounding the hospital only through the newspapers. Significantly, she was not scared off by what she read.

Einhorn interviewed her but took no action. In fairness, he had much on his mind in August of 1970 besides hiring new attending physicians, but a space was available in the department and Dr. Rodriguez's qualifications were superb. Yet her application lay dormant for more than two months. She had a cultural legitimacy at Lincoln that he did not. Her youth and stated interest in the community would appeal to the Collective. Finally, Dr. Rodriguez's specialty was his—the newborn. Her presence on the staff could set up a clinical competition in the inner sanctums of his domain that may well have been unthinkable to him. Yet Einhorn was perceptive enough to know that he didn't have objective grounds to turn her down. Had he refused a well-qualified Puerto Rican pediatrician admission to his staff in the midst of the controversy about his leadership of the department, and had the information leaked out, the wrath of the Collective, the community, and the community board might well have crushed him. So he temporized.

Fortunately, Dr. Rodriguez had also applied to Albert Einstein

College of Medicine. Drs. Fraad and Barnett interviewed her, liked her and eventually came to see her as an alternative to Dr. Einhorn. Late in October they informed us of her existence and we sent a group to meet with her. It was hard not to be drawn to her. We called her Helen from the outset because she felt like one of us. She had spent the better part of the previous decade in Puerto Rico working medically and politically for the welfare of the poor and for the equalization of the standard of living. She had become an "Independista"—one who believes that Puerto Rico should become an independent nation. Returning to New York for family reasons, she saw her place as working with poor Puerto Ricans in the city. She felt that community control was the only long-term hope for upgrading services received by minority communities from city institutions. She was familiar with the concept of collectivism and understood our desire to work in that way. Her presence felt comfortable from the start.

Early in November we were told by Dr. Fraad that an agreement had been worked out with Dr. Einhorn whereby Dr. Rodriguez would join the Lincoln staff as the assistant director of the department. At the end of the transition period—perhaps a month—Dr. Einhorn would resign his post at Lincoln, maintaining his faculty rank and status, and move elsewhere in the Einstein complex. The plan seemed reasonable to us. It let everyone off the hook and it allowed the Pediatric Department at Lincoln to move ahead with its basic mission —patient care and teaching—and to pursue the more experimental aspects of the new program initiated by the Collective. Significantly, it provided Dr. Einhorn with a new assignment with no diminution in salary or rank.

Einhorn didn't see it that way. For him Lincoln was not a job; it was a creation, a part of his being. He had no desire to make a simple academic trade. When Dr. Rodriguez attempted to assume her post in early November, he snubbed her repeatedly, refusing to acknowledge her presence in the department. Moreover, he continued to dicker with Einstein over the terms of his departure. After a week or so of indecision, Einstein recalled Dr. Rodriguez, suggesting to us that they had no intention of following through on their agreement. I can remember being furious. We had worked in limbo for months, our department was a shambles, our new programs stillborn, and a solution was clearly at hand in the person of Helen Rodriguez. Yet Einstein balked. Until that time the Collective had taken no formal position on Einhorn. It was widely and accurately accepted that we favored Dr. Rodriguez, but we had avoided taking an official stand because of disagreements within our own ranks about the appropriateness of such action. Now everyone was incensed and we easily agreed to leaflet the hospital the next morning. Stridently worded, the leaflet was entitled "Einhorn Must Go." We listed what we considered to be his failures as director and announced the existence of Dr. Rodriguez. "The Pediatric Collective demands," we concluded, "that Dr. Einhorn be removed and that hospital workers participate in appointing the new Director of Service."

Beyond its importance to us I doubt that the leaflet had much impact on the hospital or the medical school. Then on the evening of November 16th the *New York Post* carried a front-page story headlined "Fire Lincoln Hospital MD as Ethnically Unqualified." The article triggered a fire storm that was to last for more than a month. Without identifying its sources, the *Post* claimed the existence of a "statement" acknowledging that Einstein was replacing Einhorn "because of political reasons. The Dept. of Pediatrics finds it essential at this time to have a director of different ethnic background." Subsequently the *Post* revealed that the "statement" was actually a letter signed by Dr. Labe Scheinberg, dean of Einstein College of Medicine. In other words, Dr. Rodriguez was to replace Dr. Einhorn because she was Puerto Rican and he was Jewish. The story had even stronger impact because Einstein is a medical school sponsored by Jewish philanthropy. The notion that such an institution would dismiss one of its own on racial grounds in favor of a Puerto Rican was dynamite in a city where a quarter of the population is Jewish. And Einhorn knew it.

The initial story in the *Post* was quickly followed by prominent coverage in New York's other papers quoting the same document. These articles were followed by a wave of journalistic inquiries into just what was happening at Lincoln. The papers tended to characterize the situation as a confrontation between "radicals" and a dedicated pediatrician who had been inexplicably "overthrown." At one point *The New York Times* ran a biographical sketch of Dr. Einhorn, billing him as a Resistance hero who had devoted his career to the care of poor children. Who, the sketch seemed to ask, could possibly quarrel with such a man? And inevitably the *Times* and the *News* came to Einhorn's defense editorially, deploring the racism and weakness of Einstein and the insubordination of the pediatrician's underlings—the Collective. Alone among the papers, the *Post* attempted to explore the many facets of the situation that led to Einhorn's dismissal. But even then the intricate questions of community control and departmental leadership tended to pale beside the electrifying and intriguing fact of an apparently racial firing.

And that, to those of us who knew the Lincoln situation well, was the most perplexing and disturbing question. Where had the issue of anti-Semitism come from? Who had publicized it and why? In all the strife and factionalism that had taken place at Lincoln, Einhorn's racial identity had simply not been an issue. Numerous real issues separated the Collective and Einhorn, the community and Einstein, the radicals and the forces in control at Lincoln. But suddenly the entire city was buzzing over an issue that was not and never had been at stake at Lincoln. Obviously, in 1970, after ten years of civil rights struggle in the United States, everyone was sensitive to the aspirations of inner-city communities. Open admissions, community control, busing for racial mix were all current issues in New York. Indeed, by 1970 Lincoln had a number of black department directors and Puerto Rican administrators suggesting the growing recognition of racial awareness by the city and the medical school leadership. But neither the Collective nor any of the community groups that had agitated for control at Lincoln had ever demanded Einhorn's ouster because he was Jewish. Yet that was the issue that brought much of the city to his defense.

At first we doubted that the much-quoted document alleging "political" and "ethnic" consideration in Einhorn's dismissal existed. We were told subsequently, however, that Einhorn had received a letter from Dean Scheinberg of the medical school stating that his departure from Lincoln would in no way be a reflection on his medical abilities. The dean unwisely included the verbatim wording of a Pediatric Department memo on the subject of Einhorn. The letter proved to be a gun, loaded and cocked. It did not take Einhorn long to fire it.

Although the accusations of racism implicated the Collective, the principal target of the new war was the medical school. That made sense in Dr. Einhorn's battle scheme since it was Einstein and not the Collective or the community who could reinstate the department director. His only hope was to embarrass the school so badly that they would be forced to support him and, presumably, dismiss the Collective. And embarrass them he did. The city was fascinated and perplexed as to why a Jewish medical school, supported by Jewish philanthropy, devoted in large part to the training of Jewish physicians should turn on one of its own and dismiss him for ethnic reasons. The Jewish Defense League responded immediately. They stormed Dean Scheinberg's office; they picketed, sat-in, and issued a series of furious press releases demanding reinstatement, "reparations," and the like. The Human Relations Commission of the City of New York announced a full-scale investigation of the situation at Lincoln. New York's Jewish newspapers railed against the anti-Semitism and the "Nazi police state tactics" used against Einhorn. The media, in general, deplored Einstein's bad judgment and supported Einhorn editorially.

Nothing, of course, had changed at Lincoln. Nothing really had happened to precipitate this massive crisis that had the city so concerned. But the concern was sufficient to generate a great deal of activity on the part of the medical school and the Health and Hospital Corporation. Neither organization could dismiss the crisis. Einhorn's document existed and could not be explained away. Yet the reasons for removing him from Lincoln loomed clearer than ever. Reinstating him would have been both an admission of guilt and an invitation to more trouble at Lincoln. Despite the devastating repercussions of Einhorn's assault, his strategy was doomed to ultimate failure. His charge of racism with its semblance of authenticity generated great quantities of sympathy for him throughout the city. But it garnered him little substantive support because it was an essentially hollow charge that had little to do with the reasons he was in trouble at Lincoln. Einstein, though embarrassed, remained resolute in its decision that he must leave Lincoln. The Health and Hospital Corporation, satisfied that racial outrage was not really the issue, supported the medical school's position. And Einhorn, for his part, had no fall-back positions. Editorial support, city commission studies, and Jewish Defense League sorties could not change the basic situation at Lincoln. Einstein quietly moved to enforce its initial plan. Einhorn would be "reinstated" for a period of time (agreed to be about a month). Dr. Rodriguez would be retained as the associate director of the department. Sometime in December, Dr. Einhorn would take a leave of absence from Lincoln, going to Europe on sabbatical. He would receive his full salary, which would be charged against the Lincoln budget. Dr. Rodriguez would take charge of the Pediatric Department and, on his return to New York, Dr. Einhorn would be placed elsewhere in the Einstein complex.

Surprisingly, events followed the agreed-upon pattern. Einhorn was seen very little at Lincoln for the remainder of his "tenure." He did leave on sabbatical and when he returned some months later he was put in charge of clinical pediatrics at Jacobi Hospital. Dr. Rodriguez took over the department and started the hard task of stabilizing the old program in order to build a new one. The public, by and large, was left in a state of confusion. The newspaper accounts of the "re-instatement" followed by Einhorn's departure made no sense to those who understood Einhorn to be a Resistance hero wronged by a malicious anti-Semitic hand. When the evil hand seemed to have its way in spite of exposure, many people were incredulous. The problem, of course, was that the press had focused on only a small and unrepresentative part of the whole story. Some months later the Commission on Human Relations finished a detailed inquest into the situation at Lincoln that included dozens of interviews at Lincoln and Einstein. They concluded that racism had not been the issue in the Einhorn situation and closed their files on the case. Einhorn had lost, the Collective has survived. And as usual at Lincoln, there was no real winner.

The "offing" of Einhorn, as we came to call it, was an event that the Collective neither sought nor foresaw. We did not come to Lincoln with the quiet intent of removing the chief of service. Certainly there were some outspoken members of our group who called for his ouster early on and others who considered it a triumph when it happened. Most did not. What happened between Einhorn and the Collective was not by design or cunning; it was more biological than it was political. His system and ours were simply incompatible. He was impossibly authoritarian while we were outrageously antiauthoritarian —facts neither of us appreciated sufficiently at the outset.

As I sat down to write this account of the events that led to his departure I had planned to stage a hypothetical debate between him and me to dramatize our differences. I got as far as an outline of the discussion when I realized what a dull debate it would have been. On most issues we agreed: more city money for Lincoln, more status for Lincoln within the Einstein system, American house staff for Lincoln, emphasis on social medicine, outreach where possible, and on and on. We would have argued hard over community control but even that would have been more a question of personality than politics. Einhorn would not have been against community participation but he would not have chosen it for *his* department. Ultimately, it was style and demeanor that separated us and that did not make for a very good debate then or now.

Einhorn's departure from Lincoln proved to be a paradoxical event for the Collective. We were satisfied that we could finally pursue our new program without constant warfare within the department and we were delighted to have Dr. Rodriguez as our leader. But quietly the ante had been upped. To many observers we had become a group of mutineers who had captured their troubled ship, dismissed the captain, and set sail themselves. The question that flowed from that analysis and that dogged the Collective for the rest of its existence was, "Can you do a better job than Einhorn?" That was a question we had never intended to answer. The Lincoln Project as it was conceived and the Collective as it emerged were never designed as an alternative to Einhorn. His departure, to be sure, freed us in many ways but it also burdened us. It invited us, it beckoned us to show that we could "run" Lincoln Pediatrics in a better fashion than he could. To many critics it forever placed us in the shadow of Einhorn. Mostly, in fact, it left us with a badly disorganized, understaffed department, an uninitiated new chief, and Lincoln's same old problems. We were hardly victorious.

9

After the Fall

The departure of Einhorn effectively ended the first six tumultuous months of the Collective at Lincoln. We had been embroiled in a number of acrimonious battles and had received a great deal more public exposure than we had ever anticipated. The problems we faced changed markedly when Dr. Rodriguez took over. The resistance mentality we had adopted during the early part of our tenure at Lincoln was no longer relevant. Our job became to support Helen Rodriguez and to rebuild the department in a way that made it more responsive to and more involved with the community. That was a task made more difficult by the conditions after Einhorn's departure. First of all, the foreign medical graduates in the department, loyal to Einhorn from the start, all departed with him. Their defection represented almost a 25 percent loss in house staff in the department and made coverage of the basic pediatric chores (staffing the Emergency Room, night coverage, and so on) far more difficult. Moreover, many physicians in the Einstein complex felt that Einhorn had been badly treated and that we were to blame. A number of pediatric sub-specialists who served as consultants and teachers subscribed to that interpretation and refused to come to Lincoln to lecture. Many others were upset or scared by the negative publicity and let it be known that they would prefer not to be required to spend time at Lincoln.

Fast on the heels of Dr. Rodriguez's takeover we realized a growing sense of isolation. Our teaching program was in shambles. The omnivorous demands of patient care set against our depleted staff consumed much of our energy. Einstein provided no additional interns or residents to supplant those who left with Einhorn, so we were forced to pay the price of institutional turmoil with our own lives. We all spent extra nights on duty and pulled additional shifts in the Emergency Room to cover the vacated slots. Ironically, our Community

Elective Program which should have flowered under the new leadership almost ceased to exist because elective time had to be canceled so that we could meet the basic requirements of in-hospital care. Many of us felt cheated by the turn of events. It seemed we had swapped chaos for travail.

Dr. Rodriguez lent us some perspective on the situation. She described the first days of the University of Puerto Rico Medical School in the early sixties. She had been a student and a resident in the initial years of the program. They were poor, lacked prestige, faced heavy patient care demands, and still succeeded in building a good program. Many of us believed that to be an attending physician one had to have years of specialized training and experience. Not so, she argued. She told us of her classmates who had passed directly from the ranks of the house staff into the teaching positions so key to a training institution. Careful attention to academics, the diligent use of journals, and frequent attendance at conferences could more than make up for the pedagogic defections.

Cuba, too, was a source of inspiration. We knew that the island nation had lost almost one-half of its physicians at the time of the revolution. Allied with Batista by ties of class and privilege, they had fled their country to escape Communism. Ostracized by the North American medical community and subject to a punitive embargo that included drugs and medical supplies, Cuban physicians had held the line against disease and initiated a remarkable resurgence in health care. A decade after the revolution there were almost twice as many doctors in Cuba as during the fifties and indices of medical care such as the infant mortality rate and adult longevity had improved dramatically. This argued to us that medical workers with unpopular ideas could endure and, in time, prevail.

There was, of course, a major difference between the Puerto Rican or the Cuban situation and ours at Lincoln. Impoverished or depleted as those systems were, the leaders in Puerto Rico and Cuba were at least in control of the resources available. They were in charge of the systems they proposed to renovate. Helen Rodriguez was not. Lincoln and Lincoln's Pediatric Department remained on the rack between Einstein College of Medicine and the City of New York. The final decisions on budget, staffing, renovations, and direction did not reside in the South Bronx. They had not under Einhorn (who at least possessed the grudging respect of the medical school) and they did not under Helen Rodriguez. She had the power, she quickly learned, to shift things around in the department, but she had relatively little say as to what came into the department. She was tethered to the Lincoln "realities" as defined by Drs. Joe English and Labe Scheinberg.

The time following Einhorn's departure saw a number of important developments for the Collective. We had been so embattled during the first six months of our time at Lincoln that coordination and program within the Collective had scarcely been defined, let alone refined. The relative quiet that followed December of 1970 allowed us to begin to structure and rework our program as we should have from the start.

We decided, for instance, that the large Collective meeting held every Tuesday evening, while valuable for disseminating information and making policy decisions, did not allow interaction, criticism, and support to take place among Collective members. Smaller groups were necessary for this. Additionally, we hoped to initiate a program of political study where we could start to learn some of the political and social facts not taught in our traditional educations. The smaller groups were essential for this as well. Therefore, we decided to meet in one large group every second week and in small groups the intervening weeks. We divided the Collective into six sections with eight to ten members in each.

The small groups were a refreshing contrast to the cumbersome and contentious large group sessions. Issues were indeed debated in a much fuller and more intimate fashion. We read and discussed a great deal, focusing on the Chinese Revolution and its impact on health care. We read Mao, haltingly passing the Red Book in Chinese fashion from person to person for each new quotation. We wrestled with the question of what it was to *serve the people* in the context of America and the South Bronx. We learned to respect the tremendous importance of what Mao called a person's "practice" as opposed to his rhetoric or his posturing. This, of course, had implications for the Collective. Who, we found ourselves asking, were the talkers among our numbers and who were the doers? Were there not also many individuals outside our ranks whose stated position did not agree with ours but whose dedication and consistency to medical care at Lincoln made their practice exemplary?

The internal developments of the Collective had much more importance for us than they did for the community. We recognized this and knew that the real test of our precepts lay in the magnitude and effectiveness of community input into the department. The Collective assigned Paul Bloom and myself the task of organizing a Pediatric Parents Association. Working with several people who had been active in "Think Lincoln," we began our effort. The idea was simple but, as far as I know, unprecedented. Most schools, public or private, have a Parent Teachers Association (PTA). The purpose of that group is to keep the parents informed of developments at the school and give them some forum for input into school policy. The amount and style of input varies greatly from school to school but the principle is a sound and relatively uncontroversial one. Hospitals simply do not have an analog to PTA's. Why not, we asked ourselves? Two reasons occurred to us immediately—one supportable and the other not. The more understandable reason had to do with the relationship between the clients and the institution in the two situations. School is a major and ever-present concern in a parent's life. Five days a week, nine months a year, the child spends a major portion of his waking hours at school. The involvement is inescapable. A hospital is different. Indeed, health services in general are different. They are, usually, a sometime thing. When they are needed they rank as extremely important in the life of an individual or family. But when good health prevails their need is only hypothetical and they are easily forgotten or given low priority in family concerns. Thus the impetus to remain involved with the hospital is often not present. To us that was an acceptable—though lamentable—fact of life.

The second reason for citizen apathy concerning the institutions of medical care was, we felt, an inappropriate and unnecessary belief in the mystique of medicine. Most parents have been through school and, reasonably, feel they might have something to say about their children's education. They are not cowed by the classroom or by teachers. Hospitals and doctors are a different question. Many patients feel that they don't have the training, the technical knowledge, or, perhaps, the *chutzpah* to deal with the institutions of medicine. They know what they like and don't like in terms of doctors, costs, and waiting time but they somehow feel they don't have the capacity to get involved; they don't expect a role. Put simply, there is little patient demand for involvement in the administration of hospitals. This stands in marked contrast to other institutions of our society such as schools, churches, and police departments.

Our notion of a Pediatric Parent Association (PPA) aimed to

counter both of these problems. We hoped to develop a group of parents who would relate to the Pediatric Department on a continuous basis even though they would probably need to use it as individuals only occasionally. We intended to educate them in the department and its problems so that they could begin to speak with some authority about conditions at Lincoln. For a two-week period we passed out flyers to hundreds of parents in the clinic and Emergency Room waiting areas asking them to join the parents' group for a lecture and a discussion. Our efforts were met with both interest and disbelief, enthusiasm and querulousness. In any event, about twenty parents, mostly mothers, arrived for the first meeting. Paul and I served cookies and soft drinks and I thought to myself, "Shades of Mississippi and the Freedom Democratic party." "We Shall Overcome" with a Latin beat seemed in order but we had no singing. We gave a brief talk on lead poisoning as a community problem and then turned the meeting to a discussion of forming a permanent group. Dr. Rodriguez dropped by to welcome the parents and assured them that there was a place for them in the department.

Somewhat awkwardly the group members began to talk among themselves. They did not know each other. If they knew anybody, they knew us, the doctors. They were divided about evenly between blacks and Puerto Ricans. Several of the latter did not speak English and none of the blacks spoke Spanish. In spite of these obstacles the group elected officers, listed medical topics they wanted to learn more about, and agreed on a date for the next meeting. Over the following months the Pediatric Parents Association met biweekly, heard a number of medical lectures, and toured the hospital area by area. Each week after the meeting we would visit a different section of the pediatric domain interviewing the people working there and detailing the omnipresent problems. About ten parents came regularly and many others visited once or twice. The accomplishments of the Pediatric Parents Association startled no one. Generally quiet in their style and modest in their demands, they supported the medical staff in efforts to block budget cuts at the hospital, they participated in the selection process for new house staff, and they added a legitimacy and a direction to a number of departmental decisions.

The participation of the Pediatric Parents Association in the selection process for new interns and residents was perhaps their most concrete activity. Traditionally house officer training programs are fiefdoms run at the discretion and in the style of the program director. Einhorn was somewhat more autocratic than the average department chief, but his uncontested exercise of power within *his* bailiwick ranked as commonplace in medical school departments. In this tradition most section bosses singlehandedly pick their own interns and residents. Occasionally a trusted member of the department or an enterprising chief resident are included in the interviews or have a say in the selection process. But in almost all cases, the boss makes the final decisions. The house staff does not shape itself and the community served by the hospital has no say whatsoever about the doctors being hired to serve them.

The notion, then, that the community have a voice in the selection process was a major departure from tradition and it was a partial and significant fulfillment of our goal of community participation in the department. The PPA assigned three of its members to work on the selection committee. They joined like numbers of the house staff, nursing staff, and attending staff to form the complete committee. The group decided on the interview format and conducted its own evaluation at the end of all sessions. Their final task was to rank all the candidates they had interviewed, listing their strengths and weaknesses. Dr. Rodriguez made the final selection with the guidance of the committee rankings. The mothers from the PPA spoke up right from the start, often asking tough questions about applicants' attitudes toward blacks or Puerto Ricans. Interestingly, the group frequently arrived at unanimous opinions regarding the people they interviewed. This in no way meant that the parents did not have significant impact on the process. Rather it suggested that when subjected to the battery of questions from medical staff, nonmedical staff, and community representatives, the pros and cons of each candidate tended to appear in a similar light to all judges regardless of bias. The process seemed to us a significant improvement over the routine internship interview, since it provided Dr. Rodriguez with information and opinions that would not normally have been available to her.

I am sure there was an impact of our unorthodox screening system on the candidates, although this was even more difficult to assess. Surely the experience said something to them about the nature of life in the Pediatric Department at Lincoln. If they found it disquieting or degrading to be interviewed and judged by people other than their medical peers, Lincoln Pediatrics was clearly not for them. If, on the other hand, the egalitarianism of the process appealed to them, the interview probably meant more than all the rhetoric they had heard and brochures they had read.

In an interesting session late one afternoon we had a child conduct the interview of a surprised but game candidate. We had a set of three questions that we asked every candidate about his or her background, interest in Lincoln, and knowledge of Lincoln. We took turns asking these basic questions. The PPA representative had arrived with her ten-year-old son who had been shopping with her and whom she didn't want to send home alone after dark. The boy was attentive and bright and followed two interviews with interest. Somebody made a joke about his running the third session and suddenly it seemed like a good idea. The boy was eager to try and we wrote out the questions for him. He read them clearly in his fifth-grader's voice to the medical student who sought an internship in the coming year. The student responded well, occasionally asking the boy to clarify a question. The Puerto Rican youth did so accurately and unflinchingly. At the conclusion of what turned out to be a good interview we asked the candidate what he thought about the process. He admitted that he had been nonplused at first at being quizzed by a child. But as the conference progressed and the group proved to be friendly he felt he could open up and talk a little bit about himself. On balance, he stated, it was by far the most provocative and instructive of his many internship interviews.

The PPA was, in sum, a quiet effort to extend some measure of medical franchise to a large community that enjoyed very little say in its health care. At Lincoln, as in any hospital, there existed a second important community that, likewise, exercised little control over the direction of the hospital—the nonmedical staff. Obviously the kitchen workers, the nurses, the clerks, the orderlies and the elevator operators didn't have the same problems, style, or expectations. Moreover, in New York all of these groups had strong unions and at least had their say in work conditions and salary. But their power extended no further than their labor negotiations, and tradition dictated that those negotiations concern the workers only and not patient care. "Management" decisions were made by the hospital administration and, to a lesser degree, by the medical staff. Clearly we could not offer the workers a greater role in the hospital administration, since we did not have that to give. But we could greatly increase the participation of the non-medical staff in decision making on a departmental level. To do that we had to begin talking first to the other workers in the department. Each area within the department (the Emergency Room, the Out-patient Clinic, the wards, and the nurseries) had a tripartite staff —medical (interns and residents), nursing (including aides or order-lies), and clerical. Separated, more or less, by background, education, sex, and race, each staff had a separate hierarchy and reported ultimately to different bosses—the doctors to Dr. Rodriguez, the nurses to the director of nursing, and the clerks to the hospital administrator in charge of clerks. Moreover, the multiple divisive factors haunting the health care team in any section of the hospital were exacerbated by the relative permanence of the nurses and clerks and the constant rotation of the house staff.

So it was that we had to begin by talking—attempting to establish some regular form of communication between ourselves and the nursing and clerical staffs. Things went badly from the start for at least two reasons. The first was suspicion: doctors had never particularly sought the opinions or the involvement of the nurses, aides, and clerks before. Why should they now? The second was politics. Each staff had a pecking order of its own and many people—especially the higher-ups —resented the threat to the autonomy of the individual staffs suggested by meetings across the lines. We proposed fortnightly get-togethers in each pediatric area to discuss common problems and attempt solutions—a benign enough concept. But not so at Lincoln. The head clerk considered forbidding the clerical staff from attending. The head nurse in pediatrics insisted on showing up at every meeting in spite of the fact that we carefully explained to her that we wanted direct interchange between the people working regularly in an area. She talked incessantly and had a chilling effect on the rest of the nurses.

Other problems developed as the meetings progressed. We asked that the nurses and clerks be honest with us and feel free to criticize doctors as they felt appropriate. This was clearly a tough challenge for workers taught not to express open opinions about doctors. Given the chance they either found it too difficult and remained mute or, occasionally, burst out in a bitter and, usually, unconstructive attack on an individual. On our side we did little better, rarely articulating many negative feelings we all harbored about certain clerks and nurses. Things became still worse after several months of meetings when a number of problems had been clearly identified in each pediatric area but not rectified. For instance, in the Out-patient Clinic the nurses constantly complained that the doctors arrived late to see their patients. They went so far as to clock everyone one week to prove that almost everybody came late. We agreed with their criticism and promised to try to arrive on time. We announced the problem at Pediatric Department meeting and at Collective meeting and urged people to be less tardy. But there were almost forty members of the department attending clinic at one time or another. All had various chores to do before clinic, and some people took the nurses' demand less seriously than others. No major change in the arrival pattern of the medical staff resulted from our "open" and "honest" discussions and the nurses and clerks became more cynical than ever. A facade of openness and flexibility, we learned, was more destructive than no flexibility at all.

Before the meeting scheme collapsed completely we stumbled on a method of communication that salvaged the idea in part and promoted some important, ongoing communication between staffs. Obvious in retrospect but elusive at the time, medical education ("in-service training" as the nurses called it) was of interest to everybody. In fact, due to the poverty of the education program for nurses at Lincoln and the complete absence of one for the clerical staff, people were hungry for information about the diseases and problems they saw daily in their work. One morning at a particularly slow meeting in the Out-patient Department an aide complained that her TB test had turned positive and was itching her. She showed it around. The topic caught on quickly. It turned out that almost half the nonmedical staff had positive TB tests but few had any clear understanding what that meant. Some thought they had TB while others thought they were "weak" from TB and were likely to come down with it. We thoroughly discussed TB testing—a procedure done fifteen or twenty times a day in the clinic—and moved speedily on to a discussion of TB itself. Interest ran high and when time was out people volunteered half a dozen other topics that they would like to cover. The experience was the same in all the areas of the department. Medical topics fascinated the staff because the subjects related to them as people concerned about the illnesses and also as workers called on to treat patients with the conditions. Furthermore, health education came as a gift from the medical staff—something we could supply and which the administration had not seen fit to program for their workers. It had an inherent honesty and poignancy which promoted communication, interest and, in the long run, improved care in the hospital. Our hapless worker meetings were replaced by frequent health education sessions in all parts of the department. The agenda of team work and worker democracy was well, if belatedly, served by the recognition of health education as a major arena of communication in the department.

The months following the troubled summer of 1970 saw developments at Lincoln in areas other than the Collective. The activists of the community mental health strike who had become the core of "Think Lincoln" underwent yet another metamorphosis. They formed the Health Revolutionary Unity Movement (HRUM). The new organization broadened its goals to encompass a revolutionary platform for reform in the medical system. Moreover, the activists in the South Bronx joined forces with similar groups at several other hospitals in New York to form a citywide movement. While there were some whites involved in the group, its focus was Third World—black and Puerto Rican. Its ideology and practice drew increasingly from the Chinese experience with emphasis on disciplined collectivism. HRUM published a regular newspaper, *For the People's Health,* calling attention to the inconsistencies and injustices suffered by workers and patients in city hospitals. They practiced democratic, non-hierarchical relations among themselves, calling for other workers to do likewise. In summary of their views they issued a ten-point program:

1) We want community-worker control of all health services in our oppressed communities.
2) We want the right to form organizations of patients and workers to fight for improved working conditions, better patient care, and to make health policies.
3) We want all new hospitals currently under construction to be built immediately to serve the needs of our oppressed communities.
4) We want full employment and upgrading for our people in all health facilities and open admissions to all health schools.
5) We want free health care for all people.
6) We want community-run health clinics on every block to deal with minor health problems.
7) We want door-to-door preventive care to deal with sanitation control, nutrition, drug addiction, child day care, and senior citizen services.
8) We want educational programs that expose the leading health problems such as unemployment, poor housing, racism, malnutrition, police brutality, and all other forms of exploitation.
9) We want community, students, unions, and workers' organizations to actively support and fight for this program in the interests of our people.
10) The role of the Health Revolutionary Unity Movement is to educate and unite all our people and to expose the corrupt health system that keeps our people weak and unable to fight for self-determination and complete liberation.

HRUM used every opportunity to publicize its program in the belief that the strength of the ideas would popularize them. Far and away the boldest new concept in the ten-point program was the community-worker emphasis. Virtually all previous agitation in the area of institution control had invoked the concept of "community control." The notion that the work place belongs, to some degree, to those who work there was new. Additionally, this concept recognized that at Lincoln the worker and the community had much in common and that they should not be pitted against one another but should work together against their common antagonists. Many of the programs that took root in the Pediatric Department were predicated on this concept. The PPA, for instance, was involved with hospital workers in making plans and decisions within the department. Both were serving in that way for the first time and they found much common ground. The formal Community Advisory Board for the hospital functioned very differently. When members of the board were invited to join with the administration to screen applicants for the hospital director position which again fell vacant in the fall of 1971, they refused pointblank to invite any hospital workers to join them. They used every argument from ignorance to untrustworthiness to oppose the inclusion of workers. Their opposition proved more a commentary on themselves than it did a reflection on the workers' abilities. The men and women of the board did not receive their medical care at Lincoln. The result was that the board shared much in common with the administrators and the bureaucrats and was innately suspicious of the workers, an overwhelming majority of whom came from the very community that the board purported to represent. The real patients and parents who worked within the Pediatric Department had no trouble in establishing a commonality with the workers from the department. The strength of workers and community together stood as a threat to entrenched forces who sought to use the hospital for their own ends. The development and articulation of the worker-community concept was much to the credit of the HRUM.

An interesting and constructive outcome of some of the medical and political criticism that had been rained on Lincoln was the involvement of the Pediatric Department starting in 1971 with a group known as the Community Medical Corps (CMC). Initiated several years earlier by two Einstein medical students, the CMC had obtained city funds to run a small door-to-door health screening program in the South Bronx. The money was used to hire and train eight community residents who actually carried out the apartment-by-apartment medical testing. In 1971 the community workers and the students had a falling out over the management of the program and the workers turned to Dr. Rodriguez for help. They asked that Lincoln Pediatrics take over the effort and serve as their fiscal agent. Dr. Rodriguez agreed and assigned Charlotte Phillips to work half time with the CMC doing training and supervision.

The stated intent of the CMC was lead poisoning detection, since the funds obtained from the city were for that purpose. In fact, the program was much broader than that in concept and execution. The CMC workers were trained to take blood pressures, draw blood, apply TB tests, and collect urine and stool specimens. They functioned in the community as general medical screeners, looking for signs of disease and arranging follow-up at Lincoln when they found it. They worked methodically, mapping out the area north of the hospital and moving street by street and building by building, often taking several weeks to cover a block or two. They attacked some of the worst, decaying, lead-encrusted, rat-infested housing in the city of New York— Kelly Street, Fox Street, Hoe Avenue, and others like them. Three days a week they would visit new apartments, usually in pairs, a man and a woman. At these first visits they would explain the program, offering TB tests to everyone and anemia and lead poisoning blood tests for the children. They would then apply the TB (Tine) test and arrange a return visit in two or three days. On the alternate two days a week they would return with a Collective member to the apartments already visited. They would read the TB tests and draw the necessary blood. (The physician was present to provide supervision and legitimacy although it was our long-term plan to eliminate the physician altogether. Applying and reading TB tests and drawing blood—even from young, squirming children—are skills that a well-trained technician can do easily.) The CMC did its own follow-ups, arranging hospital visits for all positive or suspicious results. Generally they were well received. Families were surprised and delighted to get some medical attention in their homes. Little distinction was made when I traveled with them as to who was doctor and who was not. Children, of course, didn't enjoy getting stuck for blood, but the CMC bag included an ample supply of lollipops. They did about as well as any pediatrician in making amends.

One afternoon when I was working as part of the team, we drew blood from two particularly uncooperative small children in a crumbling apartment. We were tired, the mother exasperated, and the kids angry. One of the CMC workers was squeezing the blood from the second child out of the syringe into the rubber-capped test tube that would be used for the trip to the lab. He was hurrying and pushing hard on the plunger to get the blood to pass into the test tube more quickly. Suddenly the end of the syringe gave way and a jet of dark liquid shot out of the syringe and across the room. It splattered on the younger child who sat eating his lollipop and all over the family's couch. It was a low moment for the CMC. The child started to scream again, the worker barked some bilingual epithets, and the mother ran to clean her couch. We left promising not to take any more blood and she assured us everything would be all right. I am sure that today somewhere in the Bronx there is still a dingy couch with a great brown arc described on it, a monument to our work.

The CMC was a locally based, highly relevant attack on several of the major medical blights of slum neighborhoods. It cost little, spent its budget on the community, in the community, searched out real, treatable problems, and produced results. It was also politically expeditious. The city funded the program when it did because lead poisoning had become a troublesome problem and the Department of Health had money for "innovative" lead-detection programs. Lincoln had also been nettlesome and noisy for the city. A little money for the troublemakers, the reasoning doubtless went, would be oil on water. The program received city support through 1973. At that point lead was no longer as explosive an issue and Lincoln had been relatively quiet. The CMC was dropped and the city's apparent commitment to door-to-door medical care, its fleeting micro-assault on lead, anemia, and TB, disappeared.

The time following Einhorn's departure was important because the viability of the Collective and its ideas was being tested. Practice rather than theory, implementation rather than rhetoric became the essential components of the program. Working in informal alliance, the Collective, HRUM, the Pediatric Parents Association, and the CMC tried to put their precepts to work. Occasionally successful, frequently frustrated, the groups labored to alter the course of the hospital. At times the results of their efforts were determined by their own discipline and commitment. More often the facts of life at Lincoln continued to be governed by the medical school, the city and the society as a whole. Inertia, neglect, and decay proved potent adversaries in the fight for change.

10

Philosopher-kings or Workers

The innovations undertaken by the Collective, HRUM, and the Pediatric Parents Association changed many elements of life at Lincoln. Many of us believed that we were participating in a new age at Lincoln and that, perhaps, our experiences would prove a blueprint for renovation at other blighted public hospitals. As time passed, though, and we grew to know and understand Lincoln better, our earlier headiness and optimism began to pale. The stalemate at Lincoln was real. It was the product of forces and standoffs that, in some cases by accident and in some by design, ordained the paralysis and decay that were Lincoln. These situations were not beyond challenge or change but they were, in many instances, well beyond our influence.

There was, for instance, the trade-off between the city and the medical school: adversaries on many issues, frequent deft critics of one another, the two administrations fell into step and marched smartly in common defense against assaults from outside the hospital. Moreover, the mere presence of two administrations stood as a marvelously effective Catch 22 against change. A fugue state existed around the many undeniable areas of hospital malfunction, the city blaming Einstein, Einstein shrugging and pointing its finger back at the city. To rectify some nursing problems, for instance, the city authorized the medical school to hire a number of nurses as part of its large annual contract. Traditionally the Nursing Service at Lincoln was staffed and paid directly by the city. Given the conditions at Lincoln, Einstein felt it could not hire and retain nurses at the city pay scale so it adopted one of its own, offering, in essence, a bonus for working at Lincoln under the medical school. They succeeded in hiring the allotted number of nurses but soon found themselves under fire for abusing the established city pay rates. The city nurses protested that they were suffering discrimination and the city accused Einstein of misusing contract money. The result: Einstein dropped the bonus, the new nurses quit, and the status quo emerged victorious. It is not an accident that General Motors, the Mayo Clinic, and the Cinicinnati Reds run and run well under a single set of managers. Lincoln's twin administrations were a stone around the neck of efficiency, accountability, and change.

Then, too, there was the problem of the community. Although we frequently talked about "Lincoln's community" or the "South Bronx community" we learned quickly that the 350,000 or so denizens of the South Bronx were anything but one community. Racially disparate, linguistically divided, its populace was isolated, cornered, alienated in countless social, economic, and ethnic ways. The usual factors of poverty, decay, and racism were complicated by isolation, racial mixture, and an economy that sent people scratching over the five boroughs of New York in search of work. Nobody claimed with any measure of pride or well-formulated anger that they came from the South Bronx as they might from Harlem or Bed-Stuy or Watts or Hough. When, in the mid-sixties, the lids were regularly blowing off ghetto neighborhoods, the South Bronx could only muster a little gang warfare as its contribution to the general protest. Lincoln's community boasted no Martin Luther Kings, Bobby Seales, or Imamu Barakas. The only politician of much note associated with the area is Congressman Herman Badillo and he neither grew up nor lives in the South Bronx.

Countless factions competed for power and purported to represent "the people." Block bosses, ward heelers, political clubs, street gangs, dope runners, poverty pimps, and church leaders vied for followers. The problem with virtually every community group was that their *raison d'être*, their common cause, was themselves and their narrowly defined membership rather than any broadly defined South Bronx community. With the plethora of groups and a general absence of communal definition, the task became difficult for us or anyone else trying to open the hospital to community direction and criticism. Our quarrel with the city over its selection of the hospital's official Community Advisory Board was not that it should have been easy for them to select a better group but that the board they selected was slanted in a narrow fashion to complement and support their own positions. Their board was nonpatient, professional, and anti-worker in character. That also was the complexion of the city administration and, as such, the two groups tended to work well, if not particularly productively, together.

The real measure of a well-organized community, of course, would have been an attack on the conduct of the hospital and of the Community Advisory Board by elements who saw accurately that medical care was not being well served by the city–Einstein duumverate. That assault, in fact, developed. "Think Lincoln," the Young Lords, and HRUM, armed with facts, incidents, and medical staff sympathy, took on the hospital hierarchy repeatedly for more than two years. These groups distinguished themselves from the feuding ghetto elements that surrounded the hospital by their broad definition of the community and social struggle and by the relative absence of personal aggrandizement in their ambitions. Unfortunately, their base was relatively small and their goals and strategies different enough from the typical factions so that they attracted partisans only with difficulty. Their energies and devotion were considerable but over time they were no match for the injunctions, police cordons, arrests, bad press, and foot-dragging used against them.

If there were problems of administration and community well beyond our influence that stymied the development of the Collective at Lincoln, there were also essential problems inherent to our group that created difficulties for the growth of the program. First among these was the existence of two simultaneous tendencies in the Collective—political reform and cultural rebellion.

What brought the Collective to Lincoln and gained it notoriety was a political revolt against the prevailing medical system in the South Bronx. Politics—the politics of health care and the politics of the prevailing American urban system—were very much on the minds of Collective members, both as a group and as individuals, during our time at Lincoln. But political dissent was only part of the challenge that the Collective represented. A second revolt—in some ways more consistent and more potent than the political one—marked the entire life of the Collective. It was a personal revolt, a cultural rebellion, a statement of protest against the white-coated uniformity, the stodgy affluence, the self-serving hypocrisy, the racist and sexist narrowness of the medical establishment. That revolt called for new allegiances and priorities, experimental life styles, new modes of dress and sexual behavior. Born of the youth rebellion of the sixties, the ideas were new and particularly iconoclastic in the context of medicine, where the rule had been conformity in dress and behavior as well as clinical practice. Some people joined the Collective with a much clearer sense of individual oppression and personal revolt than others, but no one remained untouched by it. For a long time I resisted the thought that the Collective was anything other than a purely political assault on the system. And yet as far back as medical school, when I became involved in the SWAB campaign to save Waller's beard, I was part of a growing attack on the drab and sometimes dictatorial culture that surrounded medicine.

From the first thoughts of the Lincoln Project our aims were political. "However different our political orientations may be," we wrote in the initial recruitment brochure, "we share a common sense of the need for political change in effecting real changes in an environment which now generates disease." Our clearly stated, if ambitious, intent was to change the system for the delivery of medical care in the South Bronx. This was an unabashedly political goal. Yet our political efforts at Lincoln were launched at the very time when the Movement politics of the sixties were splintering. The Student Health Movement, our ideological progenitor, was virtually dead. Civil rights had long since passed on as a binding issue, while the war drove people to varied expressions of resistance. Women's rights, worker power, and Gay Liberation had growing constituencies. Violence and sectarianism had increasing currency. Endowed with experience and rhetoric from the past, but set against the turbulent and schismatic political landscape of the early seventies, the Collective began its political life.

We were the New Left in medicine. Subjective, principled, angry, often arrogant, we felt no ties with the past. We weren't Communists or socialists, we were "radicals." We tended toward isolation, avoiding ties with any number of medical and political reform groups. Even the SHO and MCHR drew as much criticism as support when they were mentioned at Collective meetings. Significantly, we did ally ourselves with the Panthers, the Lords, and HRUM, which gave us a stronger and more visible political stance. Yet relations with the first two largely amounted to their accepting our money and occasionally asking us for support in an action. Only with HRUM did our alliance have real substance. Their platform asked worker-community control of health institutions with an increasing demand for "Third World" (black and Puerto Rican) leadership. Those positions made sense to us. Moreover, they functioned as a collective. When they began to work with us, I found their emphasis on the teachings of Mao too catechismal. I felt silly sitting in a circle reading quotations from the

Red Book and passing it on. In time, though, I found Mao's writings and HRUM's discussions of service, practice, and collectivism relevant and helpful in my day-to-day experience. Under their tutelage we read William Hinton's *Fanshen*, Edward Snow's *Red Star Over China*, and a number of pieces on the American labor movement. Their emphasis on consistency and service provided a stabilizing and positive influence on the Collective.

But even with HRUM—perhaps most graphically with HRUM— we found ourselves following others and failing to define an actual politics of our own. HRUM asked that we "take leadership" from them because they were a Third World organization and, therefore, had a legitimacy at Lincoln that we did not. We accepted, partly in agreement with their principles and partly, I feel, for lack of alternatives of our own. Their leadership stressed the need for discipline in both political learning and political action. In 1971 HRUM split into two collectives—HRUM for Third World activists and the Health Revolutionary Alliance (HRA) for whites dedicated to their cause. HRA's major activity, as it developed, was to work with the Collective. HRA, in the scheme of things, "took leadership" from HRUM and, in turn, "gave leadership" to us.

It was really HRA members—usually white radicals employed outside of Lincoln in some health field—who attempted to give cohesiveness and direction to the Collective through 1971 and 1972. They attended and often led the small group meetings of the Collective, prescribed readings, conveyed requests from HRUM, and participated in Collective decision making. While I personally agreed with their estimate of the need for Collective discipline and I respected the many hours of diligent effort they spent on the Collective, I couldn't help resenting somewhat the imposition of an outside discipline—an unpopular public position but one that I think many people felt on one level or another. The radical response at the time to my objection about taking leadership from those who were taking leadership was that liberal white intellectuals were so elitist and so individualist that if they (we) were to be part of a people's movement they would have to shed their traditional decision-making role and accept the direction of the people—HRUM.

All in all, the arrangement with HRUM, which lasted for the better part of two years, told a great deal about the politics of the Collective. As with so much of the New Left, our criticisms were stronger than our platforms, our objections sharper than our remedies. We were, I think, incisive and morally correct in our criticisms of the medical care offered the people of the South Bronx, but between some small reforms within our own department and some quixotically grand slogans for the society as a whole, we had very little in the way of a political program. As a group we knew very little history, eschewed the Old Left entirely, and were outrageously suspicious and territorial about most contemporaneous political groups. The result was that the Collective confined itself to important, but relatively apolitical, inter-departmental reforms and finally with a degree of desperation embraced somebody else's politics, those of HRUM.

There was an additional element in our relationship with HRUM. The word *guilt* was much used throughout the late sixties and early seventies as a term of critical derogation. The left accused the center of being "guilty liberals" while moderates were busy labeling activists as "guilty radicals." The idea that guilt was an inappropriate, weak, or, even sick reason for political activity enjoyed credence in all camps. An element of guilt was unquestionably present in the actions of the Collective. We denied it as a group and I know I often rejected the epithet personally when discussing Lincoln. Yet guilt was to a real degree a binding and motivating force in the Collective as it was in the New Left in general. We were functioning as the conscience of the society as a whole, advertising its shortcomings and attempting to change them. In terms of medicine this was graphically clear. New though we were to the profession, we had chosen to make a stand at an overrun, underfinanced, antiquated hospital to underscore what the system was like. But we were a part of the system in so many ways. Socially, educationally, ethically we were virtually indistinguishable from the medical profession that had let Lincoln—and the hundreds of Lincolns around the country—come to be. On some level, as much as we belabored the differences between ourselves and the profession as a whole, we recognized our similarities and that caused us guilt. I don't think it was an unrealistic or an unhealthy assessment of the situation despite the stigma that the notion of guilt called down on us. We *were* part of the problem. Different from our forebears and many of our colleagues, we hoped to be part of the solution.

Acknowledged or not, the guilt drove us to certain patterns of action. The subservience we displayed in our relations with the Panthers, the Lords and, most notably, HRUM was a good example. The system that had neglected Lincoln over the years had asserted its politics boldly and ruthlessly. It had not listened to the people of the South Bronx but rather had followed its own precepts to its own advantage. We understood that clearly and on some level felt guilty about it. Obviously we wanted to behave differently, with the result that we bent over backward not to assert ourselves but to accept the leadership of the indigenous groups. So it was that the Collective didn't object to giving the Lords regular financial support without any say in their organization or activities, and officially nobody minded when HRUM turned us over to HRA for leadership without our being consulted. In a sense it was guilt wed to the principle of community control that allowed us to function smoothly in support of the community groups during their period of strength. That same guilt, though, prevented us from further defining our own politics in a way that would give us strength in the absence of HRUM, the Lords, and the Panthers. That failure contributed significantly to the demise of the Collective in the ensuing years.

While the leitmotif of guilt found throughout the politics of the Collective was in many ways beneficial to our efforts when directed outward, it tended to turn acrid and destructive when aimed inward. First of all, we were a setup for anyone with radical rhetoric and/or affiliations with a community group of which we approved. We agreed that it was our job to lend cars to members of HRUM and the Detox Program who needed them for "political" work. It was only after numerous parking tickets, several accidents, and some not-so-political trips that even the most devoted Collective members stopped the service. For a time we were a favorite target for bail money for anyone vaguely related to the Panthers, Lords, or HRUM regardless of what offense led to arrest. At one point we landed in the middle of a feud between two rival Panther factions who wanted access to our funds. In general, we had difficulty distinguishing between appropriate requests made of us and unreasonable demands made by other radicals —Third World or white. At the large pre-Collective meeting held in May of 1970, for instance, two women rose to join the debate while we were discussing salary sharing. Annoyed as if they had been through the argument countless times, they berated the assembly for wasting any time on the issue at all. How, they demanded to know, could we pretend to be "political" and even entertain the idea that we would not give our salaries back to the community? The only legitimate topic, they held, was how to dispose of the money. Their salvos enlivened the debate considerably but when some Collective members continued to balk at the idea of a massive tithe, the two women left in disgust, never to be seen again. They were not members of the Collective; they did not intend to work at Lincoln; they offered no information about their incomes, nor did they ever indicate that they shared their salaries with anyone. They had a strong rhetorical position, the morality of which we respected. We had no tools, however, to separate the "correctness" of their position from the inappropriateness of their presentation. The result was a long and bitter debate that lasted well after they departed, got us no closer to resolution of the question, and left considerable animosity within our group.

The concepts of criticism and self-criticism became extremely popular as the Collective developed. We believed generally that people should both support and chastise each other directly. Likewise, it was felt that individuals should be open to criticism and prepared to change and grow in accordance with it. Yet this very spirit of openness and self-development (which stand as abiding and extraordinary strengths of the Collective and the New Left in general) left the doors wide open for all manner of moralistic overkill and radical oneupmanship. Criticism at times became a way of life in the Collective. "I want to criticize so-and-so for such-and-such . . ." became a standard lead at Collective meetings. More often than not it was followed—without resolution of the previous assault—by soemone else criticizing yet another party for some other deviation. Statements of chastisement always far outnumbered statements of support or appreciation. The minutes of a Collective meeting in October of 1970 suggest the flavor of many of our discussions. "The chairman [of the meeting] was criticized as rigid and somewhat arbitrary. . . . The chairman concurred . . . Hank criticizes absences and bad spirit and lack of participation. . . . Oz thinks people are too polite. . . . Chuck raises question of why we're so morose. He suggests that the next meeting be devoted to interrelationships entirely. Meeting adjourned." Criticism was wielded like a wooden bat in a traditional Oriental drama. "I am going to swing the bat," someone would announce. "I am going to swing it at so-and-so . . ." "Now I am swinging the bat . . ." "See the bat swing . . ."

Overwhelmed by medical duties, inefficient and, often, ill-directed in our political work, we became frustrated and guilty about our own inaction. Criticism of others laced with a little self-criticism became a form of release, a tonic that we hoped would cure our political confusion. The criticism and self-criticism sessions that followed every Collective meeting were so unpleasant that, I remember thinking, they must be good for something. We were Calvinists as well as Jacobins.

The failure of the Collective's political revolt and the attendant disillusionment was reflected in the Collective meeting of August 10, 1971, some thirteen months into our tenure. The minutes state that "There were present feelings of 'something missing' from the Collective this year—of dissatisfaction and frustration, of hopes unmet and actions not carried through." The anonymous scribe summarized the discussion in what he or she called "Reflective Minutes."

> Who are we
> What are we
> What are we doing
> What are we doing here
> Why are we here
> Why are we?
>
> Do we follow
> Do we lead
> Do we follow a leader
> Do we lead a follower
> Do we lead a fellow
> Do we love our fellows?
>
> Do we act
> Do we activate
> Do we react, or do we reactivate?
>
> Are we philosopher-kings or workers, acters or actors?
> Is it "we" or "me"?
>
> A consensus was reached to try again.

At the same time as the political revolt embodied in the Collective grew frustrated and weaker, the personal revolt of Collective members against the system became stronger and more appealing. Disillusioned by the magnitude of our chosen political task and the growing perception of failure, Collective members began to devote more time and energy to the personal side of their objection to society. Tackling problems of life style and personal unrest often seemed more reasonable and the goal of change more attainable after a year or two of wrestling with the politics of the South Bronx.

The roots of personal objection ran deep in the Collective. Individuality and experimentation were on the ascent among youth in

America, and the Collective was no exception. The "counter culture" was all around us and while medical students in general were more orthodox than their peers, we had all been affected by the times. Many of us had worn beards, sideburns, and long hair before such styles were acceptable in the medical community. Here and there people had challenged the use of ties or the compulsive wearing of medical whites. When we arrived at Lincoln ties disappeared quickly and almost no one donned the baggy, overstarched uniforms supplied by the city. I don't recall any formal discussion of the topic at the outset beyond the general agreement that everyone should dress neatly and cleanly. I think debate on the question of liberation from ties and whites seemed needless since they were uniformly felt to be personally oppressive and, at the least, symbols of class and guild. It turned out, though, that laxness in dress and neatness didn't always go together. It is hard to say, for instance, whether sandals are neat or a doctor in a dashiki is tidy. We didn't all agree and certainly many patients found new dress styles perplexing and even distasteful. Moreover, our own maxims of tidiness were abused. A gentle note sent to Charlotte and Marty by a friendly Einstein faculty member three weeks after we started highlighted the problem. "May I please mention one item?" he wrote. "I have noted that the overwhelming majority of patients who come to the Lincoln clinic are dressed up because they are 'going to the doctors.' Some of the house staff—with the best of hearts—are not dressed neatly. Dirty jeans, a dead cigar, a shirt only partly tucked in, smoking in front of patients. Without being stuffy about doctor-patient relations I don't think this belongs because I don't think patients want it this way." From that time on the question of dress was raised periodically in Collective discussions with virtually the same points being made on all sides of the debate—individuality vs. conformity, our need for comfort vs. the patients' expectations of a doctor, personal expression vs. tradition. Every deliberation ended with the same resolve: we could wear what we liked within reason so long as it was clean and neat. We always agreed but within weeks we were back arguing the subject. Reasonable dress, neatness and cleanliness, it seemed, were highly subjective judgments and people interpreted them variously.

More important than the stylistic revolt we staged against predominant medical mores was the incipient professional revolt embodied in the Collective. Most Collective members had been involved in the SHO and, as such, had been one of a small number of activists in their medical school classes. To some degree all of us were used to standing apart from our peers and the medical profession in general. In large part all of us took exception to the medical landscape as it lay before us—training programs, medical societies, and white-coated elitism. Lincoln seemed to be an escape from that. None of us knew where Lincoln would lead but at least, for the moment, it seemed to be away from the standard corridors of medicine (academic and private) to which so much in so many of us objected. A few people arriving at Lincoln actually were quite frank to state that internship or residency at Lincoln was for them a last chance within "the system." If it didn't work they would go it on their own or give up medicine altogether. That position proved overly dramatic and no one that I know from the Collective has abandoned medicine, but the degree of alienation from the system and the amount of anomie that that position represents suggest the extent of personal rebellion that some individuals carried with them into the Collective.

Personal rebellion took many avenues at Lincoln besides clothing style or hair length. Most concretely it was seen on a medical level. Feelings within the group ran from mild antiauthoritarianism to extreme, really rigid, egalitarianism. Einhorn, I am sure, felt that our resistance to authority was reserved for him. Certainly he caught an early and large blast of it in our reluctance to attend his teaching sessions, sweep after him on rounds, and generally honor him as the supreme Director of Service. But authority figures on all sides felt the wrath of the Collective. Not only did we take on obvious adversaries such as the hospital and nursing administrators at Lincoln, but we lashed out from time to time at potential friends who occupied positions of authority—the pediatric directors at Einstein, Dr. Rodriguez after she became Chief of Service, and members of the Collective who were judged to be ambitious or "individualist." At times I came in for a great deal of harsh criticism from some Collective members. My personal relationships at Einstein as well as my role in the development of the Collective from its inception gave me a vantage point that some people felt I used "individualistically," an obvious breach of collective function, if so. At one point in a Collective meeting the issue came to a vote as a motion of censure. The Collective voted not to censure me, but I can attest to the fiery antiauthoritarian breath of the Collective.

Egalitarian reforms in the medical routine were agreed on even before we started at Lincoln. It was decided that much of the division in duty between intern and resident and resident and chief resident was artificial hierarchy. Therefore, intern and resident schedules were made identical so that everybody had exactly the same number of nights on call, the same number of vacation days, and the same number of elective months. Difference in experience was largely ignored in favor of egalitarian function. On the ward where I was chief (or second-year) resident in July, duties were much altered. Instead of the interns taking responsibility for the primary care of patients, the patients on our service were to be divided among the team members without regard to "rank." At the end of rounds a list of chores (blood to be drawn or exams to be administered) was posted on the wall of the ward. Everyone chose random chores to be performed and returned to scratch them out on the list. Rounds themselves differed from the standard. Normally, the most senior resident leads rounds. The interns each update the team on their particular patients and keep track of new plans or diagnoses. Not us. We took turns, with the most bewildered intern often leading the group, trying to keep track of all the patients, or attempting to ask erudite questions on diseases he had never seen before. The system collapsed quickly of its own weight though various aspects of the work-sharing schemes lasted for the duration of the Collective. The notion of authority was generally disliked by the Collective and we went to extremes to avoid it where possible.

There were many ways in which the personal revolt verged on or even defined the political process at Lincoln. Our choice of collectivism, for instance, as our mode of political expression was due in large part to personal objection to traditional political forms. People simply didn't like the hierarchy and the egoism often found in more standard political structures. So we became a collective. On an even more basic level, our very attempt to be political in the context of house officership was a product of the personal objections that we had to the system. Normally, interns and residents are content to struggle through their weekly schedule and leave change in medicine or the world to others. We believed in participatory democracy and felt that it was our right as workers to be involved in the politics of our work place. So we invented a political house officership.

The final and most graphic area in which the personal rebellion at Lincoln could be seen was in personal relations. The medical and political changes we enacted did bring about a real sense of commonality and camaraderie. Working relations within the Pediatric Department were spirited and warm. Our efforts to include hospital staff outside of the doctors in the Collective brought mixed results. At the time I really felt that we had failed to make significant dents in the rigid divisions that isolate one group of hospital workers from another. Yet when I returned to Lincoln for a visit several years after all vestiges of Collective function were gone from the Pediatric Department, I was accosted immediately by a group of nurses' aides. "Dr. Mullan, where have you been? And where are all those doctors who were here with you? The ones who knew our names, and called us to meetings and took good care of the patients. Where have you all been? We miss you." At least to some degree the Collective was remembered as doctors who related warmly to patients and workers. That made me feel good.

A number of experiments in living and relating grew up around Lincoln. Three or four groups of Collective members shared large houses or apartments for periods of time. For many months a small but hardy group met at seven every weekday morning for breakfast to discuss interpersonal relations. At the pre-Collective meeting there was talk of forming a women's caucus for the Collective. I remember kidding with Judy about forming a ladies' auxiliary, a joke nobody thought particularly funny. A month or two after the Collective arrived at Lincoln, the women doctors in the Collective, several nurses, and half a dozen wives (Judy included) had formed themselves into a formal women's group with the goal of meeting regularly to discuss problems they shared as women. They met weekly for two years providing support, insight, and criticism for one another. The first group gave rise to a second and then to a third.

It is hard to tally precisely the impact of the women's movement on life at Lincoln. There were no melodramatic women's lib confrontations in the hospital. Rather, by stages men became more aware of feminist positions, of differential attitudes toward women, and of sexual undertones in the evaluation of women. The women argued, persuasively I thought, that women's issues should be given a priority within a Pediatric Department since virtually every child was accompanied by a mother and that by far the majority of the workers in the department were women—nurses, aides, technicians, dieticians, and so forth. They lobbied for the provision of adequate day care both for patient-mothers and worker-mothers, a playroom for children in the clinic area and on the pediatric wards, and available and medically sound abortion program (elective abortions had been discontinued following the death of Carmen Rodriguez), and an accessible and sensitive birth control and gynecology service. With the possible exception of the last, none of these basic services for women functioned very well or for long at Lincoln. And little was done to change that by the administration which felt that day care was the mother's problem and abortions were too controversial for Lincoln. The hospital absorbed the demands of the women's movement at Lincoln much as they did the community requests made to them. They acknowledged the veracity of the issues and then swallowed any plan for action in the twin bureaucracies of the hospital.

The women's movement did have a more permanent effect on the men at Lincoln. Within the Collective and, to some degree, in the hospital in general, men became serious advocates of the women's demands—seeing, in many cases, problems they had not even been aware of several years before. Under the influence of the women's demands, for instance, I became an expert in clinic playroom facilities, a topic never taught in residency nor examined by the American Board of Pediatrics. Working full time in the Pediatric Out-patient Clinic in my second year, it occurred to me that we had no entertainment for the dozens of children who waited for hours every day to see the doctor. I visited a number of facilities in the Bronx and saw playrooms and day care arrangements that provided marvelous service for mothers and children. After months of negotiation we got the administration to designate a tiny portion of the waiting area as a Pediatric Playroom but, at length, they balked at the provision of funds for renovations, supplies, or personnel. We did build a book rack in the clinic and kept it stocked with books and toys that we hustled from local toy manufacturers. It proved to be a popular addition to the clinic area.

From the women's movement came men's groups. One day in a hospital corridor I was approached by two male Collective members, men with whom I had sparred intellectually and politically on many occasions. "We're starting a men's group and we want you to join," announced the first. A men's group! What next! I thought, being only vaguely comfortable with the concept of women's groups at the time. "Fitz," added the other earnestly, "we think you *really* need it." That was more than I could take. I saw the invitation as an aggressive barb, a new and clever level of stag competitiveness. I turned them down immediately stating, as I recall, that if I was having problems in my relationships with women I could better spend my evenings at home cleaning house than in meeting with the boys to talk about it.

They proceeded to meet without me. In spite of my rejection of the group I was curious about it. I had to admit to being perplexed at my lack of close male friendships in recent years and at the degree of competitiveness that seemed to shroud my relations with other men in medicine. I also felt that the Collective, dedicated though it was to egalitarianism and harmony, suffered from considerable male-dominated, internecine aggression and strife. With a dim appreciation of all this and with a growing sense that the now functional men's group intended to examine men's relations with men, I joined.

Ten or so of us met weekly for more than a year. Predominantly doctors, mostly self-conscious radicals, we lamented the absence of dock workers, taxicab drivers, and cops from the group but concluded, accurately I think, that our style defined us and we had to deal, first and foremost, with who we were. At the outset rancor, oneupmanship and harsh criticism were far more common than support, warmth, and friendship. In time though, that began to change. We cooked for one another, took a Saturday trip to the beach, talked one after another about our childhoods, parents, schools, and marriages. Simple enough on the surface, the agenda led to much greater understanding and much more warmth within the group. While most people don't consider an honest rendition of their life story a closely guarded secret, it is rare for most people—certainly urban, scientifically trained, busy men—to tell their tales completely before an attentive and sympathetic small audience.

I cooked spaghetti for the group one night, leaving work early to do the shopping and to start the sauce simmering. That session a young lawyer talked about his homosexuality and how he had come to terms with it. On other occasions two group members who had been recently divorced discussed what they had been through. I missed a session because Judy had just delivered our first child, an eight-pound, five-ounce girl. (Everyone in her women's group had girls—an amazing seven in a row.) We spent the entire next meeting on childbirth and fatherhood. Judy had delivered naturally and the group was fascinated to learn what it had been like to be a Lamaze father. I was proud, enthusiastic, and only too happy to talk. Our sessions were not entirely without division and acrimony. Lincoln members in the group, particularly, tended to open old wounds from time to time and go after each other over work-related problems. Yet I found that the effect of both listening and talking was astonishing. Animosities and grudges that I carried with me into the group tended to melt as our discussions developed. I found myself comparing many aspects of my upbringing and life with those of other group members whom I had previously considered hostile or threatening. That process developed an empathy within me. I sometimes remained critical but there was a warmth and a positivism to my criticisms. After our autobiographies, we chose topics for discussion week by week in advance—marriage, sexuality, children, work, the future, and so forth.

Early on we assumed that our group would be activist and that we would undertake projects or actions of a political nature. In fact, the personal focus became so strong and so appropriate that we never developed much of a political program. We attended one or two peace demonstrations as a unit (which turned out not to be very different from attending demonstrations as a nonunit) and several of our members participated in the 1971 May Day Action in Washington, D.C., and were arrested like most people. But political action did not become our focus or, for that matter, that of any of the several other men's groups that sprang up around Lincoln at about the same time. Most of us had fairly political jobs or at least we saw them that way. Politics and political concern were not lacking from our lives. Rather, the men's group offered something quite different, quite out of the ordinary in our existence. It offered male intimacy, comparison, self-exploration in a generally supportive atmosphere. Those qualities were novel, or at least unusual, in our lives and as such gave our meetings, our unity, a poignancy quite different from political activity.

There were risks in our group structure but fortunately none of them became problems for us. The absence of a leader, and, to a degree, the denial that expertise in interpersonal affairs existed at all was consistent with the antiauthoritarianism of the Lincoln experience. In consequence, we tended to grope our way toward issues, often failing to realize when we had hit on a topic of particular meaning to one or another group member. We heard tales subsequently of individuals in similar groups who had become acutely anxious or severely depressed as a result of their discussions, while the group proved either unaware of the problem or unable to cope with it. Leaderless groups can also fall prey to opportunism with a strong or clever individual dominating the sessions for his own purposes. We encountered neither of these problems and the leaderless format offered us some real advantages. It was inexpensive, spontaneous, and truly nonauthoritarian. It helped me understand and, I think, overcome a certain amount of intellectualized competitiveness and alienation that I harbored. Simply put, it provided male friendship and support in a modern, urban life that was short on those commodities. I left the men's group when I left New York. Since then I have seen men from the group occasionally and there remains a special intimacy between us. We are at once ex-bowling partners and old war buddies; we have played together, but we have also been under fire in the same trench. Their friendship is special.

Speaking broadly, the Collective's political revolt tended toward failure while the personal one flourished. Ironically, both circumstances pushed the Collective toward dissolution. The growing frustration and disillusionment that accompanied the inability of the Collective to effect quantifiable change in the hospital or the community contributed to poor participation in Collective activities, the tendency for Collective members to leave Lincoln at the end of their contracted obligation, and the failure to recruit new physicians to the ranks of the Collective. After a year at Lincoln many interns found themselves wanting to work in a setting where they could "get it together personally"; that is, spend time with family or friends in a pleasant setting. Many Collective members began to question the degree of commitment that Lincoln required. If one's personal reflections led to the conclusion that medical school, with its demands on time and person, was an unhealthy experience, Lincoln proved worse. When medical work was completed there were meetings to be attended, flyers to be distributed, readings to be done, and street clinics to be staffed. Even standard house officerships seemed undemanding in comparison to being a political physician at Lincoln.

Recruitment became a problem. While we had easily filled all the available pediatric slots in our first year, Dr. Rodriguez found herself with fewer applicants in 1971 and still fewer in 1972. The romance was over. American applicants (political or otherwise) tended once again to consider Lincoln for what it was and not what it might become. Moreover, the nature of medical students was changing rapidly. The mood of the seventies was far more passive than that of the previous decade. Whereas a politicized, activist house officership appealed to many of us, fewer and fewer students seemed inclined toward protest and direct redress of problems. The result was diminished interest in the Collective and Lincoln among political applicants. There were some bright spots. The Departments of Medicine and Psychiatry attracted a number of house officers who came because of the Collective and Dr. Rodriguez succeeded in hiring several good attending physicians in Pediatrics who wanted to work in a political setting. But after 1970 the Collective steadily diminished in size.

During 1973 the Lords and HRUM underwent major changes. Both groups decided that workers rather than the community should be their focus and that their independent stances were not conducive to worker organizing. Therefore, the Lords became the Puerto Rican Revolutionary Workers Organization and HRUM dissolved in favor of work within unions by its members. The Panthers had disappeared from the South Bronx scene some time before. That left the Collective on its own with uncertain politics and few allies. By 1974 Pediatrics looked much as it had five years before, foreign medical graduates filling almost all positions. Some of the patient-care innovations begun by the Collective remained intact and the department continued to enjoy good leadership under Dr. Rodriguez and her successor, Dr. Evelyn Bouden. But collectivism, community control, and worker democracy had ceased to be issues. The Department of Medicine remained a focus for political medicine for some time, continuing to recruit house officers interested in social change and quietly instituting Collective reforms on their service. A handful of people—mostly from Medicine—met as the Collective through the summer of 1975, when they disbanded, feeling they could best continue their work within the context of their own departments.

I left Lincoln in July of 1972 after two years of work, the first as a resident and the second as an attending physician. The experience was rewarding and frustrating, enraging and confusing, instructive and troubling. Personally I began to lose track of what was happening at the time the Lincoln Project became the Collective. The Lincoln Project was simple, straightforward, something I clearly understood. It was an SHO Summer Project writ large. Its goals were doctor-oriented, doctor-dominated, and modest (social medicine and educational reform). Collectivism implied much more. Collectivism put revolution on the horizon. It called for a new politics among ourselves, in the hospital, and in the community. It invited massive personal self-assessment and change as doctor and as human being. It raised the specter of a new society. Collectivism was idealistic, ambitious, and perhaps most important, arrogant. It assumed success and tended to ignore or belittle those who disagreed with it. That assumption gave it the strength to set up shop quickly and with visibility, but it also tended to cast many of the people it encountered as enemies because of their adherence to the status quo. The Collective talked at length about friendship and alliance with patients, progressive workers, and radical physicians while, in fact, the majority of patients, workers, and physicians at Lincoln, for better or for worse, took exception to the politics and the style of the Collective. That fact left the Collective in an unrealistic and, ironically, elitist position from which it never recovered.

I think I felt the necessity for personal revolt less than many members of the Collective. Lincoln and the South Bronx caused me anger and indignation (much as Mississippi and medical school had) but the prevailing medical and political systems did not drive me to a sense of alienation and oppression that many Collective members articulated. And those feelings more than anything metamorphosed the Lincoln Project into the Lincoln Collective. They were powerful feelings derived from and kindred to the spirit that drove the youth revolt of the sixties, that put civil rights on the map, that eventually stopped the war. Yet at Lincoln they were bound for a dead end. The Collective's sense of alienation and oppression were simply not strong enough nor widely enough shared to build a permanent political coalition at Lincoln. As the Collective we had staked out far more medical and political ground than we could ever control. With some accuracy on all counts we found the unions corrupt and self-seeking, the Community Board irrelevant, and the Committee of Interns and Residents (the doctors' union) bourgeois. When HRUM and the Lords pulled out, we were left alone to carry out our revolution. But by then we had lost track of it in the mundane realities of life at Lincoln. Discouraged, frustrated, and politically adrift, the Collective disintegrated.

I came to Lincoln with the expectation of remaining a year or two. I had dealt with the war and the draft by obtaining deferred appointment in the Public Health Service, for which I owed two years to the government at the end of my residency. In some ways that knowledge protected me against depression; when things went badly for the Collective, I knew I had to leave anyway. In other ways my planned departure was troubling. I felt that to be consistent in my work at Lincoln I should be prepared to spend many years of my life at the hospital. Yet Lincoln was an uncomfortable place in so many ways: conditions were terrible, the work load staggering, the likelihood of change small. Those realizations were compounded by the failure of the Collective. We had such good reasons for choosing the hospital in the first place and yet our plan failed in so many ways. For much of my twenty-four months I agonized over the inconsistencies in my own logic. I had chosen Lincoln; no one forced me to work there. The work was medically vital and politically important and yet somehow unfulfilling. We made very little progress on any front and spent great quantities of time arguing among ourselves as to why not. At times I found myself thinking, "If only I had come to Lincoln quietly and joined Charlotte and David in minor internal hospital reforms . . . Would we not have been more effective and happier?"

Living in New York did not prove easy either. Judy and I shared a comfortable middle-class life on the Upper West Side of Manhattan. There was nothing particularly extravagant about our ways—except in comparison to the patients I treated all day every day. Some evenings I climbed into my Volkswagen for the half-hour struggle home through traffic, feeling extreme relief. I couldn't wait to get to our apartment to turn on the air conditioner to blot out the oppressive heat and smell of the South Bronx or to escape to some chic restaurant with Judy to forget the misery I had seen. Other evenings I left feeling guilty. What justice was there in the accident of birth that gave me a month in Europe in the middle of my work at Lincoln or enough money to buy a new car with no loans, no creditors, no layaways? Why couldn't my life at work and my life at home be somehow closer, more relevant to one another, more instructive and supportive of each other?

I never found an answer. Lincoln was cruel and kind, horrible and beautiful, hopeful and hopeless. I suppose all life circumstances contain contradictions but Lincoln, as I experienced it, became nothing but contradictions. I resolved the problem by leaving the hospital and the Collective after two years of labor and keeping my date with the Public Health Service. Departure turned out to be no exception to Lincoln's rule of contradiction. As I went to the Nursing Station in every section of the Pediatric Department on my last day on duty to say good-by I was wracked with ambivalence. "Why are you leaving, Dr. Mullan?" a nurse asked me flatly. "I owe the Public Health Service two years and my time has come," I responded mechanically. "But we need you here," she countered. How could I disagree? The simplicity of her statement underscored its veracity. Leaving Lincoln resolved my conflicts about the Collective and it allowed me to fulfill my commitment to the government but it did nothing to help the people of the South Bronx—a cause to which I had been firmly devoted for more than two years. I felt unhappiness and not relief as I bade my farewells to staff members, workers, and patients.

I think now I was too hard on myself when I left the Bronx. It is true that in many ways the Collective was a failure. Certainly we did not achieve the sweeping changes in medical care that we had hoped to when we first came together. Yet we had made an honest stand for what we thought was right and worked hard in support of it. That many of us perceived the failure and eventually moved on did not mean that we were unprincipled or irresponsible. The more telling personal question for me and the other members of the Collective was, did we remain faithful to the radical precepts that brought us to Lincoln after we left or did we burn out, drop out, or slip back into the mainstream of medicine? Put differently, was our challenge of the early seventies shallow and faddish or did it represent an episode, a chapter in a consistent personal effort to change medicine and society?

That is not a question that can be answered simply or definitively at this time. I think, though, that Collective members have generally exercised a consistency and an imaginativeness in pursuing their careers and their principles after leaving Lincoln. Despite the fact that the political and medical scene is quieter and less flamboyant than it was when we all passed through medical school and house officership, people have still managed to find meaningful medical work that remains consistent with principles developed in that earlier epoch. Let me cite a few examples.

On joining the Public Health Service I went to New Mexico in the National Health Service Corps, a new program designed to provide physicians for medically underserved areas. Assigned to *La Clinica de la Gente*, a Chicano clinic in the barrio of Santa Fe, I learned a great deal about worker-community control and community medicine. I neither wore nor owned a Public Health Service uniform, spoke only occasionally with my supervisor in Dallas, Texas, and generally functioned in a manner indistinguishable from the other local physicians —with two notable exceptions. I charged on a sliding scale (that meant an office visit cost most of our patients one dollar) and I was accountable to the clinic's board. Major administrative decisions (fee schedules, office hours, building renovations, hiring policies, etc.) were initiated or approved by the board while medical policy and medical practice were left up to myself, the other staff physician, and our clinic nurse. Our staff worked well together, seeking out and treating more than our share of social and family problems. Once we arrived at the local hospital for a conference on one of our patients with the clinic nurse and two outreach workers as well as myself. The man suffered many medical as well as personal problems that we wanted to clarify prior to his discharge. The orthopedist who had treated him in the hospital arrived at the meeting and promptly picked an argument with a member of the visiting Nurse Service who was also present. After a round or two of acrimony, the orthopedist got up and stalked out. As he pushed out the door he growled, "I'm not going to practice medicine by committee and that's all there is to it." We practiced a lot of medicine "by committee" and it proved good for the patients and good for us.

Many of the concepts that never came to life at Lincoln worked and worked well in the community clinic setting. In fact, they hardly seemed revolutionary; they seemed sensible. Staff education, for instance, was a must. Our outreach workers had not had any medical training prior to their employment at *La Clinica*; they had to be taught. Our nurse was a local woman just out of school. Instructing her in screening and diagnostic techniques enabled us to see more patients. She has now gone back to school, perfected her skills, and rejoined the clinic as a nurse practitioner. The Community Board (all of whom were clinic patients) naturally directed the program since they had founded it. Numerous issues that had produced only heat and labels ("radical," "pig," "troublemaker," "bureaucrat") in the Bronx resolved themselves simply and constructively in the community setting. We were not without problems: staff meetings were sometimes long and argumentative; several staff members quit over disagreements with clinic policies; the board frequently failed to produce when it promised to provide workers or materials for clinic projects; and so on. But the format was healthy. The board and the medical workers had free and frequent access to one another, ensuring the democratic and reasonably efficient management of the enterprise. Community-worker control wasn't radical, it was practical.

Due to illness I had to leave *La Clinica* in mid-1975 after two and a half years as a staff physician. I am now working for the National Health Service Corps in the central office in Rockville, Maryland.

Charlotte Phillips has remained at Lincoln up to the present time. Working mostly as an attending physician in the clinic, she has taught pediatrics to several generations of Lincoln house officers and treated thousands of South Bronx children for hundreds of ailments. Paul Bloom left Lincoln in 1975 after three years as a house officer and two more as an attending. He helped develop and run a clinic for school problems where children who were having academic difficulty received the attentions of pediatricians, psychologists, and social workers functioning as a team. He is now working as a staff pediatrician in a neighborhood health center in Rockland County, New York, where he lives. A half dozen physicians who came to Lincoln as part of the Collective remain active in the Department of Medicine.

After Lincoln, Marty Stein spent two years in the Navy and two more as a pediatrician in a worker-controlled community health center in Santa Barbara, California. Now he works for the University of California at San Diego Medical School teaching pediatrics and community medicine. And Waller, who finally grew his notorious neat goatee into a full beard, spent four years at Lincoln as an intern, resident, and attending physician followed by a year off building a house in Nova Scotia and traveling the countryside. Now he is a Fellow in infectious diseases at Duke University. Like Stein and Waller, a number of other Collective members have combined academic positions with community medicine activities. Henry Kahn spent two years at the Center for Disease Control of the Public Health Service in Atlanta before joining the Satellite program of Atlanta's Grady Memorial Hospital. He also teaches in the Department of Preventive Medicine and Community Health at Emory University School of Medicine.

Following two years at a radical community clinic in the San Francisco Bay area, a husband and wife team from Lincoln moved to Chicago, where she teaches pediatrics at Cook County Hospital while he works on a masters degree in industrial medicine. Another Lincoln couple moved to Kentucky where they are living in a "hollow," raising a family, practicing medicine, and working with progressive local organizing groups. Two men who left the Collective after the first year traveled to Seattle where they have both worked part-time in a federally supported pediatric clinic and part-time in a neighborhood free clinic. And at least three graduates of the Collective are practicing medicine in the South Bronx at two different government-funded health care centers.

I have lost track of a number of Collective members and, obviously, the final *curriculum vitae* isn't in on any of us. But significantly, I can't point to anyone who has abandoned the principles of former years; no one I know of has gone into private practice, no one has accepted a medical school appointment without some community or social medicine commitment, and no one has quit medicine. Virtually everyone is practicing the skills learned at Lincoln and struggling to make them politically and personally relevant, given the institutions and opportunities available today.

And what of Lincoln Hospital? At this writing (spring 1976), a new plant for the hospital has finally been built. Eighty years after the first one, forty years after a new one was called for, twenty-five years after Jacobi borrowed the funds, and ten years after the city made a new Lincoln a "priority," the new structure is ready for business. Located fifteen blocks northwest of the present buildings, the new hospital has 700 beds—more than twice as many as the old Lincoln and a number more appropriate to the needs of the South Bronx. The city, however, has announced the imminent closure of two other municipal hospitals in the Bronx (Morrisania and Fordham), making the new Lincoln's statistical load at least as bad as that of the old one. In any event, the new facilities are reported to be good and that will do a great deal to improve hospital care in the area. Ideally, that means that there will be no more beds in the halls, no more hopelessly clogged toilets or infant "diarrhea rooms." Additionally, the new plant will make Lincoln a more appealing hospital for staff, students, and potential medical school affiliates. It may still be the poor sister of the Einstein complex but at least it has a stylish new set of clothes.

Lincoln's essential problem, however, remains. It is a latter-day charity hospital, an historical fact which neither the Health and Hospital Corporation with its computers nor Einstein College of Medicine with its academic veneer have altered. The Collective, on balance, failed to move Lincoln beyond its charity heritage. A new plant will improve patient care, but Lincoln's basic disenfranchisement within the larger system of private medicine will remain intact. It will take more than a few years of work by progressive physicians and community activists and more than the happy circumstance of a new building for the hospital to separate Lincoln permanently from its nineteenth-century origin as the Home for Worthy, Aged, Indigent Colored People.

11

My Butcher
Doesn't Believe I'm a Doctor

While I was working at Lincoln, Judy and I lived on the Upper West Side of Manhattan, a polyglot neighborhood, now rich, now poor, always interesting, sometimes rough. Near our apartment, on the ground floor of a decaying tenement destined for "urban renewal," we discovered a fabulous butcher shop. The owner, like his butcher father, was a throwback to the turn of the century. He sawdusted his floor, sported a straw hat, nipped as he worked, and knew his many customers by name. He invariably scribbled roasting instructions on the red-brown butchers' paper in which he folded the meat. He was a small businessman in the best and most traditional sense.

Learning one day that I was a doctor, he inquired with interest as to where I practiced. I explained that I worked in a city hospital and had for some time. He appeared incredulous. No matter how I described my job he had trouble grasping the concept, repeatedly inquiring as to the whereabouts of my *private* practice. "All doctors have private practices," he assured me. "That's where they see *their own* patients." I assured him that I had no private practice and that I intended to keep working for the city. He was stumped. I just didn't quite fulfill his notion of what a young doctor should be and that bothered him. Finally, he determined that I worked at a hospital with interns and residents, and, relieved, he asked me to bring him my card when I finished "at school" and did open my private office. "Lots of people in here need doctors. If you leave me your card I can see to it that you get lots of business, lots and lots of business."

My butcher had decided that doctors were businessmen, like himself. They were perhaps better educated and wealthier than he was, but, at heart, they were like him, shopkeepers. He had difficulty understanding a physician in any other way. I could not argue with him; many doctors (especially those of his generation) were just that. Yet many doctors of my generation were not. Certainly it was clear that I was not the businessman-physician that he envisioned, and I knew numerous young physicians whose style and chosen manner of practice would not conform to his sense of what a doctor was or should be. That fact didn't mean that the butcher was hopelessly out of touch; rather it argued to me that the profession had broadened in recent years, and that significant numbers of doctors were beginning to practice in ways that would have been unlikely or unacceptable in the past.

When I began practice in New Mexico, the Community Board of the clinic asked that the clinic's doctors wear white jackets or smocks to make it clear that they *were* doctors. Their reasons were two. First, we looked youthful and dressed casually and didn't much resemble the traditionally clad local physicians. Second, in the past, poor people frequently had been seen and treated by medical students, and the board wanted it clear that we were "real" doctors. Again, not only our style, but our mode and place of practice made us different from the average physician. The Community Board understood that, and appreciated it. They suggested we wear white, not in a spirit of obeisance to the medical profession, but in the recognition that patients—particularly older ones—might need help in adjusting to a community clinic with young doctors. The white coats were to be a gesture to the conservatism they anticipated in their own people. That gesture acknowledged that a generation gap did exist in medicine and that some patients, like the butcher, would find it bewildering. I happily complied, though, over time, I discovered that it didn't make much difference. Finding it hard to believe that a physician would see them in a remodeled café for a dollar a visit, they still asked me if I was a real doctor.

When I lived in New Mexico, a friend of mine became ill while visiting New York. He called me long distance to ask where he could get medical attention. I gave him the names of two excellent internists on the staff at Lincoln, and subway directions to the hospital. My friend stands six feet, six inches tall, has a full beard that hangs over his chest, and hair to his shoulders. He is always clad in a shabby blue overcoat that reaches to his ankles and resembles a relic from a Napoleonic campaign. He does not look like Marcus Welby. When he returned from New York, cured, I asked him about his visit to

Lincoln. He was delighted with the medical care he had received, but remained perplexed about the hospital. In the hour or so that he waited in the Emergency Room, two patients and an orderly had approached him, and addressed him as "Doctor," asking questions about medical problems. He mused that it was absolutely the only time in his entire life that he had been mistaken for a physician. At Lincoln, these days, the only people who look the way doctors used to look are drug company salesmen.

During most of the sixties, and part of the seventies, I assumed that I was part of a revolution. My sense and definition of that revolution developed and changed over time, but throughout, I anticipated that some sort of new order was being established in society in general, and that I specifically was involved in the retooling of medicine. Furthermore, I took the groups that I worked with to be the institutions of the revolution and fully expected them to survive and grow. Perhaps I am overstating the case slightly; I was never literal or dogmatic in my belief in change. But I certainly thought that the "Movement," as we so often and so imprecisely called it, would alter America and, to some degree, capture it.

Now I find myself asking what happened? My simple assumptions of the past years have not held up well in the mid-seventies. When reminiscing with Steve Cohen about Mississippi, or Bert King about the SHO, or Charlotte Phillips about the early days at Lincoln, I can briefly rekindle the simple belief in movement, or change, or revolution, that we shared. Yet today, that belief seems dated to me, naïve, simplistic, unserviceable, and I am left wondering, what really happened? Was there a revolution? What was accomplished? Was I a revolutionary? And toughest, who am I now?

From an orthodox point of view, it seems to me that no revolution took place. No governments were toppled. Big business, big universities, and big medicine remained intact. Ten years later, the Administration in Washington is, if anything, more conservative than it was during most of the sixties. We seem no closer to socialized medicine or even national health insurance. Worse than that, the institutions that I knew best have all vanished. The SHO and the Collective are gone. MCHR still holds periodic meetings, but it bears little resemblance to the organization that sent me to Mississippi or marched with Martin Luther King. SNCC is history, as are the Freedom Democratic party, the Lords, the Panthers, the Yippies, the Moratorium Committee, the Peace and Freedom party, and Eugene McCarthy. The organizations of radical reform generally failed to establish themselves in any long term way; by and large, they proved far more effective at protest and challenge than they did at organization and constituency building. The "Movement" turned out to be just that—movement rather than a new party, a new way of life, or a revolution.

And yet there has been change. The war was finally stopped. Civil rights and racial equality gained a permanent place on the American political agenda, winning new respect and material well-being for many people. The women's movement has emerged resolute and articulate. Medical schools are significantly more progressive than they were a decade ago, and the profession is beginning to reflect it. On balance, the ideas of the sixties fared far better than the organizations, with the "Movement" achieving a number of its goals in spite of its apparent demise. Maybe a revolution did take place, I find myself saying. Maybe it is too traditional, too Old Left, to look to the politicians or the corporations for evidence of some new order. Perhaps the revolution has already occurred in minds and spirits around the country and I missed it looking, as I have, for some concrete transfer of power, some new "ism."

The problem eventually reduces itself to semantics: what does one mean by revolution? At times my sense of revolution calls for dramatic events, people in the streets, armies on the move; while at other times I see it more subtly—new sensibilities, altered life styles, quiet personal commitments. The format of the events of the radicalism of the sixties conformed more to the former, while the outcome of the actions was the latter. The demand for change came on brash and confrontational; yet the change that resulted turned out to be temperate, frequently undramatic, and often personal. America, in the end, was not turned around as we so intensely hoped, but the course of many of her institutions was significantly altered. Was that revolution? I suspect not. But it was change, movement, important movement, and in that I do feel a small sense of pride and accomplishment.

I can be most specific about the change in medicine. We did succeed in creating a generation gap: the younger members of the profession look and act differently from their elders. That, of itself, is no particular triumph. I am quite clear now that there is no intrinsic value to long hair as opposed to short hair. Rather the importance of the change in medicine is that the profession is no longer so uniform, so monolithic. Medicine today has room for people who want to work in ghettos and on reservations, who like to smoke dope and live collectively, who prefer salaries to fee-for-service. More important, medical schools are now training more blacks, women, Chicanos, Puerto Ricans, and Indians than ever before. They will all bring their varied styles and backgrounds to bear on the profession, opening it further. More physicians today are salaried (working for universities, the government, and prepaid plans) than ever before. Fee-for-service private practice is no longer the standard for American medicine, as shown in the dwindling membership of the AMA. Partly reflecting progressive changes in medicine, and partly determining them, the political organizations of young people in the profession are quite different from what they were a decade ago. The Student American Medical Association succeeded in institutionalizing a number of SHO programs (notably the Summer Projects) and captured and preserved a fair amount of the spirit of dissent and reform of the sixties. In recent years they have been far more outspoken and activist than they were previously. Of late, they have changed their name to the American Medical Student Association (AMSA) to establish a distance, once and for all, from the AMA. On the house officer level, collective bargaining has emerged as the tool of interns and residents seeking improvements in patient care, as well as economic gains. Whereas New York's CIR stood alone as a voice for house staff in 1965, almost every city in the United States that employs interns and residents today has a vocal house officer association. Increasingly, young physicians see themselves as public employees. It is not by accident that the Physicians National Housestaff Association has allied itself with the American Federation of State, County and Municipal Employees, a union representing public employees in many fields. Young salaried physicians identify in many ways with the aspirations and problems of other hospital workers, nurses, teachers, and government employees.

Like long hair, the move toward unionism by young doctors is not good in and of itself. Unions develop in many ways and can fall prey to all manner of self-interest and corruption. To date, house officers have been vocal about patient care, hospital staffing, working hours, and working conditions which I think bodes well for the creation of a progressive labor movement in medicine. Regardless of the exact nature of the emergent unionism, the collective format is something quite new among doctors. Over the years it is true that the AMA has functioned as a (usually effective) lobby for doctors' self-interest, but the AMA has always taken care to separate itself from the common laborer. As long as they have both existed, organized medicine and organized labor have been at the opposite ends of the American political spectrum. Now a significant group of young physicians is embracing labor's strategies and accepting their support and guidance. That circumstance taken alone suggests strongly that the future of organized medicine will be quite different from its past.

Even without a political label, the new directions in medicine add up to an important new situation. The middle-aged, conservative, free-enterprise, anti-government, anti-labor hegemony in the profession no longer exists. Ten years ago it was not strong enough to prevent the passage of Medicare. Today it is far weaker. The nation remains divided on what form of national health insurance to enact, but the voice of organized medicine that has been so domineering in past medical debates is appropriately faint in the present one. Most important, when the Congress finally does vote some form of national medical coverage, there will be a large body of physicians ready to accept the program and work positively to implement it. The anticipation of massive physician resistance that once overshadowed all proposals for medical reform is no longer a reality. The precepts and experiences of young physicians have left them far more open to change than previous generations. That will be significant in years to come as medicine continues to evolve.

Looking back now over the events I have described, I am quite clear on what has happened to Lincoln Hospital over the years. Though I find it more difficult to assess, I am content with my understanding of the radicalism of the past fifteen years and its impact on medicine. I am least satisfied with my insight into myself and what has happened to me during this same period. It is easier to be psychoanalyst than autoanalyst, and far easier to be a historian than either of the others. Yet it remains important to me, and perhaps to others who have been through similar experiences, to try to understand the impact of these events on the individual. Where, in sum, have my experiences as a medical radical taken me?

At some point in 1967, during the height of my SHO activity, an adviser to our student projects approached me. I liked the man, who was a dentist, well enough but found myself questioning his consistency from time to time since he ran a lucrative, high turnover, ghetto dental practice while he worked with us. Though he disguised it well, I suspect on some level our earnestness and broad criticism of the existent health care system made him uncomfortable. "Your dean and I have been talking about you," he announced. He referred to one of the associate deans at the University of Chicago who worked on our Summer Project. "We have decided that you won't be so different after all. You are a good administrator and you see the problems too clearly not to end up like us. Ten or fifteen years from now you'll be a dean or a bureaucrat or a politician just like the rest of us. You'll be part of the system—the same system you're trying to change. We're sure of it." Part congratulatory and part condemnation, I couldn't be sure if his remarks were really aimed at me or whether they were an attempted vindication of his own position. In any case, they left me with an uneasy feeling that I have reflected on frequently since that time. What does become of youthful radicals? Do we inevitably become part of the systems we try to change, or is it possible to maintain a principled distance from the conceits and sinecures that we saw so clearly and criticized so harshly in our elders?

It was not simply good press or swaggering style that made Che Guevara easily the most popular Movement hero. He was the paradigm of the successful radical first because his revolution succeeded, second because he remained defiant and militant in spite of success, and third because he died, thereby avoiding all the pitfalls of time and age. Conversely, the group most maligned by the radicals of the sixties for their alleged shortcomings were the progressives of the thirties, the Old Left. Their revolution failed, they were later (during the McCarthy period) hunted and harassed, and, above all, they kept on living, raising families, making compromise after compromise to protect their well-being. Personally, I don't think either the adulation of Guevara or the contempt for the Old Left were accurate or fair. Moreover, neither analysis speaks to our situation, which falls, I think, somewhere between the triumph of Guevara and the suppression of the Old Left. In society in general, and in medicine in particular, we did post some victories, but on the whole we have continued to live, largely unsuppressed, in an era when progressive change seems less likely. Many of us, perhaps most of us, are over thirty, that once magical line that our youth chauvinism carved for us, and we are neither policing the streets of the nation's capital in jeeps and military fatigues nor are we locked away in slave labor camps. We are ex-youths, many of us, pursuing our lives in a mildly reformed America wondering if we are ex-radicals.

And that brings me back to some very hard questions about myself.

In the past ten years I have worked in Mississippi, practiced medicine in the South Bronx, lived in Woodlawn, marched with Martin Luther King, broken up an AMA convention, shared my salary, and picketed more often than I can remember. I took part in those events because I believed in them, and I am very glad I did. Yet I also participated because I was young and unencumbered, and risking my life in Mississippi, or living uncomfortably in Woodlawn, was relatively easy. Now things are different. I have two children, two cars, and a house. My income and my life style are indisputably American bourgeois. I find myself thinking more about the future than I used to, and in a different way. The future used to be a time for some vaguely defined fulfillment of my idealistic expectations—a time when things would be better and fairer. Now the future is more personal and more worrisome, an epoch filled with concerns about schools for the kids and income for the mortgage payments. The future seems finite now. It used to stretch forever, but now, if I'm lucky, it contains two, three, maybe four decades. That sense urges me to move on, to make compromises if necessary with my purist notions in order to achieve some degree of success, some taste of victory.

I do not mean to suggest that all radicals of the sixties have evolved as I have. Many old friends of mine lead far sparer material existences than I do and continue to be involved regularly in organizations of protest, while others have grown totally apolitical or completely self-seeking. In medicine many of us have had an easy, if seductive, route into the profession. Our medical licenses, first of all, have guaranteed us employment with good income. Second, the notoriety that we achieved has generally opened rather than closed doors for us, so that becoming part of the system has been almost unavoidable. Many of us now labor away at establishment jobs content with what we are doing, but nagged by a sense of not doing what we were supposed to be doing or, worse yet, perhaps doing what we were not supposed to be doing. Since the alternatives seem to be more of the same, we continue our efforts at medical school reform, government administration, prison health or city hospital improvements, and wonder with varying degrees of enthusiasm if some day there really will be a revolution.

If that seems like a bleak picture, I don't really think it is. Ours was a youth revolt and not a true social revolution. We protested in tandem with blacks, with Puerto Ricans, with women, and to some degree we were successful. But now we are veterans, refugees of an earlier period. And like all refugees, life is not simple for us. We are torn between adherence to our earlier culture and adaptation to the new one. In that sense I don't think we have done badly working to consolidate the gains of earlier actions and waiting, hopefully, for the emergence of a new politics, a new social consciousness that will again allow us to become activists. The obvious hazard to this simple analysis is that we will become comfortable with the present order, successful within it, and disinclined to change it further. Age does tend to temper radical spirits. I have seen it in others, and I admit to feeling it within myself. I can only speculate about the future, but I think that there remains alive within me—as within others—a spirit of objection and resistance that is the essence of radicalism. That spirit regularly and religiously points to a job unfinished, a task wanting completion. It coexists gingerly with my recognized credentials, reminding me constantly, if politely, that systems, institutions, and people are often not what they appear to be, that truth exists at the root, the *radical*, of any situation. It calls not so much for a single solution to problems (medical, political, or social) as for a process, an ongoing approach to life.

I suspect as I grow older that my radicalism will be tested in a new way. Unlike the past, where often it presented me with direct physical clashes (street marches, police confrontations, Mississippi threats), it promises to challenge my complacency in the future. As young people reach adulthood, or as today's students become interns and residents, they may well begin to make demands of me. They, or future generations, may well challenge my life style or medical practice. Workers or blacks or women, or some new unrecognized minority or oppressed group, may take exception to me or my identity (male, white, doctor, middle class, whatever), and I will be called on to respond. Will I be defensive, reactionary, self-serving, arrogant, pig-headed, or will I listen and identify as I might have in the past? I don't mean to suggest that any challenge that is mounted is *a priori* valid and therefore deserving of support. Rather, the consistency of my radicalism in the future may be tested more in how I react than in how I act. Will I be open to new ideas and movements as they develop, or will I remain fixed in the past and jealous of my own small terrain? Paul Dudley White, Benjamin Spock, and Quentin Young stand out in my mind as three physicians I encountered in my youth who have passed the test. All were successful, and all three were the recipients of society's benefits, yet all maintained a perspective on medicine and America that enabled them to be critical and continue to work for change. That test awaits our generation. The flamboyance of our youth is over. We have still to prove that we can maintain our critical outlook and our sense of objection as we move ahead in life.

I suspect that my dental friend would be satisfied with the predictions he made about my future in 1967. To him it would seem, reasonably enough, that I had settled down to the relatively staid personal and professional life that he foresaw. I don't think his prophecy has been fulfilled as simply or completely as it might seem. Significantly, my butcher doesn't really believe I'm a doctor—at least not a doctor as he or many Americans understand a doctor. Somehow I am different. For him, it was the way in which I practiced medicine that made me suspect. For others it might be my beliefs or my style of dress or my political allegiances. But for many people I have not been, and am not a doctor in the old mold. That, more than any single reform or innovation, has been my experience and my offering as I have grown up in medicine.

Some day my butcher—or his children—may grow to feel differently about medicine. They may come to appreciate the changes that are occurring, and perhaps they will again want to refer patients to me, this time not because it is good business, but because it is good medicine.